MIND, BODY, AND HEALTH
Toward an Integral Medicine

MIND, BODY, AND HEALTH
Toward an Integral Medicine

Edited by
James S. Gordon, M.D.

Depts. of Psychiatry and Community and Family Medicine
Georgetown University Medical Center

Dennis T. Jaffe, Ph.D.

Dept. of Psychiatry
UCLA School of Medicine

David E. Bresler, Ph.D.

Executive Director
Center for Integral Medicine
Los Angeles, CA

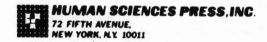
HUMAN SCIENCES PRESS, INC.
72 FIFTH AVENUE,
NEW YORK, N.Y. 10011

Printed in the United States of America
987654321

Library of Congress Cataloging in Publication Data

Main entry under title:

Mind, body, and health.

Bibliography: p.
Includes index.
1. Holistic medicine.   2. Medicine—Philosophy.
I. Gordon, James Samuel.   II. Jaffe, Dennis T.
III. Bresler, David E.   [DNLM: 1. Holistic health.
W 61 M6635]
R723.M5   1984   610   83-20159
ISBN 0-89885-150-5
ISBN 0-89885-188-2 (pbk.)

CONTRIBUTORS

Paul Brenner, M.D., University of California at San Diego; Center for Integral Medicine
David E. Bresler, Ph.D., Center for Integral Medicine
Rick J. Carlson, J.D., Health Resources Group
James Fadiman, Ph.D., Stanford University; California Institute of Transpersonal Psychology
James S. Gordon, M.D., Georgetown University Medical Center
Jan Harlow, Center for Integral Medicine; Institute for Creative Aging
Dennis T. Jaffe, Ph.D., Department of Psychiatry, UCLA School of Medicine; Center for Health Enhancement Education and Research
Dolores Krieger, R.N., Ph.D., New York University School of Education, Health, and Nursing
Richard J. Kroening, M.D., UCLA Pain Management Clinic
Evelyn Mandel, Center for Integral Medicine; founder, Institute for Creative Aging
Stephanie Matthews–Simonton, Cancer Counseling and Research Center, Fort Worth, Texas

Richard B. Miles, John F. Kennedy University, Orinda, California; Health Science Department, San Jose State University

Emmett E. Miller, M.D., Psychosomatic medicine and Hypnotherapy practitioner in California and Oahu

Kenneth R. Pelletier, Ph.D., Department of Medicine, School of Medicine, University of California at San Francisco

Robert Rodale, Rodale Press, Emmaus, Pennsylvania

C. Norman Shealy, M.D., Ph.D., Shealy Pain and Health Rehabilitation Center, Springfield, Missouri

O. Carl Simonton, M.D., Cancer Counseling and Research Center, Fort Worth, Texas

Robert L. Swearingen, M.D., Department of Orthopedic Surgery, University of Colorado School of Medicine

John Travis, M.D., M.P.H., Wellness Associates, Mill Valley, California

Michael P. Volen, M.D., formerly of the UCLA Pain Control Unit

CONTENTS

PREFACE

David E. Bresler, Ph.D.

Socially, politically, legally, and ethically, American medicine is in a state of transition. Rapid technological advances and explosive increases in scientific knowledge have resulted in rising expectations of longer life and better health on the part of all Americans. Yet, although we have witnessed the eradication of many infectious diseases and dramatic decreases in infant mortality, most Americans are not healthier. In fact, the physical, psychological, and social stresses of contemporary society continue to promote a host of acute and chronic problems that often remain unresponsive to the therapies our doctors have been trained to provide.

In Western culture, man has been conceptualized as having body, mind, and soul. This division is emphasized in the structure of our health care system: one group of professionals treats the body (physicians), another wholly separate group treats the mind (psychologists), and yet another treats the soul (clergy). While many other cultures create healing rituals that involve the whole person—and often the whole family and social group as well—our contemporary health–care system is characterized by its specialization.

Within the health–care community today, however, a new focus is emerging, characterized by an integrated approach to the individual. Treatment of the whole person—rather than treatment of the individual parts—emphasizes the psychological aspects of the healing process and stresses the maintenance of health rather than the treatment of disease. In addition, pioneering clinicians and research scientists are now seriously investigating radically new techniques that hold the promise of longer life and better health for our families and ourselves. As a result, therapeutic procedures once considered eccentric or esoteric are receiving increasing public acceptance and scientific validation. These range from centuries–old acupuncture and yoga to more modern forms of therapy such as biofeedback and guided imagery.

In treating the psychosomatic and psychosocial diseases of civilization, a variety of nonsomatic factors must be carefully evaluated. The inability to deal effectively with stress, loss, or change; problems in family or work environments; beliefs and expectations; feelings of control over one's life; self–destructive compulsive habits; and a host of problems related to human sexuality are known to affect both the onset of illness and the outcome of therapy. The enormous power of the mind has only begun to be explored, but it now seems clear that an integrated combination of mental, spiritual, and physical approaches can help to mobilize the body's intrinsic healing powers and ability for self–regulation in ways previously thought impossible. Further investigation of our inner resources may lead to even more innovative techniques for creating and maintaining health.

Practitioners of Integral Medicine are concerned primarily with people rather than disease. In their search for a common rationale that underlies all healing experiences, they view the universal life force as a benevolent process that stimulates and supports human development, rather than as an adversary which must be overcome in order to survive. Symptoms are seen as warnings that something is wrong, and the meaning of illness is explored through a therapeutic partnership in which patients and therapists share information, advice, and support.

Integral Medicine practitioners utilize individualized combinations of traditional and nontraditional approaches that maximize patient self–responsibility in the treatment process, but do not abrogate the therapist's responsibility in that process. By integrating both new and ancient concepts into the existing health–care delivery system, they are often able to offer comprehensive care to patients who have not been helped by symptomatic therapy. As a result, both doctors and patients are rediscovering the mutual trust and confidence that has traditionally been characteristic of the doctor–patient relationship.

As the trend toward specialization is becoming more balanced by the search for an integrated understanding of the life process, old rituals and new technologies are being brought together in unique and innovative ways. In the process, both are changed and the potential for total patient care moves closer to becoming a reality.

The essays in this monograph are based on presentations made several years ago at a conference on "Psychosocial Approaches to Health and Disease" sponsored by the Center for Integral Medicine and the National Institute of Mental Health. While no attempt was made to comprehensively review all of the recent developments in integral medicine, these contributions provide unique insights regarding some of the major changes that are now transforming our health care delivery system. On behalf of the Center for Integral Medicine, I would like to acknowledge our deepest appreciation to the contributors to this monograph and to Marcie Sharlott, Jack Booker, R.N., Julie Phillips, and Bob Heffron who helped with the editing, and to Judy Irsfeld, Johnne Campbell, Diane Vega, and Gloria Goldsmith who typed the manuscripts.

FOREWORD

Senator George McGovern

Modern medicine has helped bring enormous advances to the American people. Our technology and our system of health care has done much to reduce mortality from infections in the very young and the very old, to save lives that would otherwise be lost to trauma, to preserve and prolong functioning among the victims of chronic disease. It has been far less successful in helping us to reduce the stresses that lead to chronic disease and in encouraging us to change the habits—of eating and sleeping, driving and drinking—that promote illness; it has done still less to teach us how to take care of ourselves and one another.

If the title of this book tells us that its authors are moving "Toward an Integral Medicine" the essays it presents may also be seen as steps toward health promotion. In the services that the authors describe—pain control clinics, centers for runaway young people, wellness and stress reduction programs—the people who come for help begin to become aware of why they have become ill and what they can do about it.

The specific interventions that take place in these programs are diverse and at times a bit strange to a reader accustomed to pills and scalpels—meditative breathing to make it easier for an orthopedic surgeon to set a broken bone, visualization exercises to stimulate white blood cells in their fight against cancer, and family therapy to deal with adolescent physical and emotional problems. But they have two important things in common. Each helps individuals to see that they can be active in healing themselves. And each seems, at least in these early reports, to be helping people whom our orthodox medicine has little to offer, to feel better, and to take better care of themselves.

I am very pleased that the National Institute of Mental Health has had the foresight to sponsor the conference which produced these essays. We desperately need information about new directions in health care and examples to encourage us to take better care of ourselves.

INTRODUCTION

During the 1960s health–care reformers emphasized the need to extend the benefits of the medical system to underserved populations and to humanize the care that was delivered. Groups such as the Medical Committee for Human Rights declared that health care was "a right not a privilege," while Free Clinics (i.e., free at the point of delivery of care and relaxed in style) provided models of easily accessible and personally responsive primary health and mental health care.

During the last decades clinicians and researchers, policymakers, and consumers have begun to raise questions about even "the best care that money can buy" and its relevance to improving our health. They acknowledge the biomedical achievements of the last century and their contribution to the treatment and cure of a variety of diseases but question the narrowness and applicability of the model. They point out the high cost and destructive side effects of present medical treatment and its inability to stem the tide of chronic, stress–related disorders.

As this critique has enlarged and gained adherents it has set the stage for a new approach to medicine and health care. Variously called holistic, behavioral, or integral, this approach emphasizes the treatment of the whole person in his or her familial and social context and the psychological aspects of illness and of the healing process. It gives as much attention to the maintenance and promotion of health as to the treatment of disease. It fosters patient–practitioner cooperation and individual responsibility rather than dependence upon professionals.

The contributors to this volume are participants in and shapers of this new approach to health care. They have built on the work of the pioneers in psychosomatic medicine; have made clinical use of laboratory findings and electronic apparatus which demonstrate that individuals can control "involuntary physical" functions; and have begun to explore the utility of such ancient therapeutic modalities as touch, acupuncture, diet, and yoga. They have integrated these new and rediscovered techniques into the individual practice of orthopedic surgery and internal medicine, psychiatry, and obstetrics and have elaborated them in comprehensive programs for pain control and cancer therapy, health promotion, and mental health. Some have elected to work on their own; others have remained within the health–care establishment, practicing, teaching, and conducting research in medical, dental, and nursing schools.

Since 1975 the Center for Integral Medicine, based in Pacific Palisades, California, has been one focal point for those who are creating this new health care. Its public conferences, held in conjunction with the UCLA School of Medicine, have provided an opportunity for many, including the contributors to this volume, to present their work to audiences of health–care professionals and consumers.

Several years ago the National Institute of Mental Health asked the Center for Integral Medicine to organize a meeting at which clinicians and researchers, educators, and health–care organizers would have the opportunity to share and discuss work in progress. The emphasis was to be on the behavioral and environmental determinants of health and illness, on new techniques for helping individuals to mobilize their own healing capacities, and on descriptions of context for these techniques. Initial presentations were informal, personal, and speculative—progress notes rather than conclusions. Some of the contributions to this volume retain this tone. Others, revised and critiqued, carefully marshall research and clinical evidence to establish the present boundaries of the field. None, however, pretends to be definitive.

Perhaps any new approach should be granted a provisional and temporary suspension from conventional canons of evaluation. It is easier to see the shortcomings of old ways than to present certifiable programs for a new one. Time and psychic space are needed to imagine and explore alternatives to our present health–care system. An expanding, hardy critique of that system exists. We should nurture with special care for a while, the searching, tentative proposals from this new approach. From time to time we need reminding that a scientist's and clinician's job is as much the exercise of imagination as skepticism; that success lies in their tension and balance. The integral or holistic approach challenges the specialized preoccupations of a generation of dedicated medical talent. That talent brought a virtual victory over infectious diseases in developed countries. But in these countries we now have a different task of learning to control through a more integral or holistic approach the more diffuse risk factors that precipitate chronic diseases.

The arrangement of essays in this book is designed to introduce this integral or holistic approach to the reader unfamiliar with it as well as to provide an overview of the field. An introductory essay presents a perspective common to integral practitioners and offers a framework for the remainder of the volume. It is followed by a section on the capacity of the mind—through meditation, autogenic training, hypnosis, and relaxation—to control physiological functioning, and then by papers which show how physical modalities may affect both body and mind. Sections which detail the clinical practice of integral medicine, its application throughout the life cycle, and its implications for patients and practitioners follow. Finally, two essays explore the possible shape of the mental health and health–care systems that are to come.

Part I

TOWARD AN INTEGRAL MEDICINE

The essay by Drs. Gordon and Fadiman provides an overview of the clinical, social, and economic realities which have set the stage for a new, more integrated approach to medicine and a synopsis of communalities which are shared by many practitioners. It is meant to be suggestive, to whet the reader's appetite for the papers that follow and to offer a framework for approaching them.

James S. Gordon, M.D., is currently Clinical Associate Professor in the Departments of Psychiatry and Community and Family Medicine at the Georgetown University School of Medicine. He was formerly a research psychiatrist at the National Institute of Mental Health and Chief of Adolescent Services at St. Elizabeths Hospital and has been particularly concerned with comprehensive social and mental health services to adolescents and their families. More recently he has been incorporating nonpharmacological techniques in his work with people with severe mental and psychosomatic disorders. He was formerly director of the Special Study on Alternative Services for the President's Commission on Mental Health. He is author of *Caring for Youth* (NIMH, 1978) and of numerous scientific and popular articles.

James Fadiman, Ph.D., is a lecturer at Stanford University and a member of the faculty of the California Institute of Transpersonal Psychology. Dr. Fadiman is a member of the Board of Directors of the Center for Integral Medicine, a consultant to government and private agencies, and author of several books, anthologies, and articles, including *Relax* (Dell, 1976).

Drs. Gordon and Fadiman are coeditors with Arthur Hastings of *Health for the Whole Person: The Complete Guide to Holistic Medicine (Bantam Books, 1980)*.

Chapter 1

TOWARD AN INTEGRAL MEDICINE

James S. Gordon, M.D.
James Fadiman, Ph.D.

It appears to many, within and outside of the profession, that American medicine is in a time of crisis: a crisis of care, a crisis of confidence, and a crisis of costs. Though we have substantially reduced death and disability from acute infections, vitamin deficiencies, and congenital malformations during the last half century, we have done far less to stem the tide of chronic, stress–related, and "mental" illnesses which have replaced them as the chief agents of mortality and morbidity. In recent years, our medicine has begun at times to seem counterproductive and ineffective. We appear to be spending more and more money to diagnose and treat conditions that we have the knowledge to prevent, to be prescribing and submitting to surgical and pharmacological remedies which may alleviate one problem only to precipitate another.

Crisis is a time of opportunity as well as of danger. Our dissatisfaction with the quality of the health care we give and receive, and our dismay at its cost, are forcing us to look for new ways to make our medical system more humanly responsive and effective; new approaches to preventing illness and promoting health as well as treating disease; new means to help mobilize the individual's capacity for returning to and maintaining good physical and mental health. This chapter is meant to outline the dimensions of the crisis we face, to introduce some of the concepts and practices which are shaping the more holistic or integrated medical practice gradually emerging from this crisis, and to provide a framework for the clinical contributions that form the remainder of this collection.

THE CRISIS

Dollar cost is probably the single most important impetus for change in our health–care system. Between 1950 and 1977, the cost of health care accelerated at about twice the rate of all other costs. During these years, hospital charges increased from 3.7 to 65.6 billion dollars.[1] The total health–care cost for the fiscal year ending September 30, 1977, amounted to 162.6 billion dollars, or 8.8 percent of the Gross National Product, an increase of 12 percent over the previous year and an average expenditure of $737 per person.[2] The cost of individual medical care has become an unbearable burden for the 25 percent of our population who are uninsured, and it is quickly becoming one for the nation as a whole.[3]

Dissatisfaction with the quality of care given and received has risen along with its cost. During the last 15 years, our delight in the achievements of modern medicine has been overshadowed by our dismay at our inability to prevent or alleviate the chronic stress–related and "mental" illnesses which beset the anxious, overfed, sedentary, and environmentally assaulted masses. In 1974, 50 percent of deaths were attributed to cardiovascular and cerebrovascular disease, and an additional 19 percent were attributed to cancer. More than 24 million Americans have hypertension, a major predisposing factor in cardiovascular and cerebrovascular disease, and at least as many suffer from sleep onset insomnia. Ten million Americans are alcoholics, and according to the President's Commission on Mental Health, approximately 15 percent of our population "needs some form of mental health services."[4]

Until recently, the medical professions and the public alike were accustomed to taking great pride in the surgical and pharmacological treatments that were being developed for these and other illnesses. More recently, we have become aware of the shortcomings and overuse of some of our most widely employed treatments, and of the side effects that attend even judicious use. For example, studies in the late 1960s indicated that as many as 20 to 30 percent of American children had tonsillectomies and adenoidectomies,[5] but that only 2 to 3 percent of them were appropriate candidates for these procedures.[6] Several years later, a House of Representatives Subcommittee estimated that these often ill–advised and unnecessary operations were still producing "300 deaths, 15,000 operative and postoperative complications and costing 150 million dollars" each year.[7] This same report indicated that the deaths from this one procedure were just a fraction of the total morbidity and mortality from unnecessary surgery. The Committee estimated that there were 2.3 million unnecessary surgeries each year, costing 3.9 billion dollars and 11,900 lives.

More recently, it has become clear that unnecessary surgery and its lethal complications are only the most obvious examples of iatrogenic (i.e., physician– or hospital–caused) illness. Ivan Illich cites studies which indicate that one out of every five patients admitted to a typical research hospital acquires an iatrogenic disease; that one–half of these episodes results from complications of drug therapy; that one in ten comes from diagnostic procedures; and that one in 30 leads to death.[8] In a report on medical malpractice, the Department of Health, Education and Welfare estimated that "7 percent of all patients suffer compensable injuries while hospitalized."[9]

Increasingly, medical journals are reporting toxic side effects of drugs which were once considered effective and safe. Aspirin, an analgesic consumed at the rate of some 20,000 tons per year (225 tablets per person),[10] is known to cause gastrointestinal bleeding and genitourinary pathology. Librium, Valium, and Miltown, for which a 100 million prescriptions are written each year,[11] all have a high propensity for addiction and can produce severe withdrawal symptoms. The phenothiazines, a group of tranquilizers which seemed to offer great hope in the treatment of schizophrenia, have been discovered to cause a wide variety of side effects including hepatitis, leukopenia, short-term musculoskeletal abnormalities, and dose–dependent impotence, long–term disability, and a sometimes irreversible movement disorder called tardive dyskinesia. As a result, an increasing number of clinicians and investigators have begun to wonder if the cure isn't worse than the disease.

Often, physicians have claimed that the damage done by particular remedies and the settings in which they are administered, and the costs of providing them, are outweighed by their overall efficacy. However, it now seems that this contention may also be questionable. For example, in the multibillion dollar war on cancer, enthusiastic pronouncements by researchers and clinicians and the National Cancer Society must now be evaluated against the background of accumulated data. In the course of questioning the usefulness of the five–year survival rate as an "indication of progress in cancer control," Enstrom and Austin cited figures from the California Tumor Registry to indicate that "since 1950, there has been no increase in the total survival rate for localized cases (of cancer) and only a slight increase in cancer at all stages."[12] We may be less likely to die from some forms of cancer (e.g., stomach), but we are more likely to succumb to others, (e.g., lung). Even our success in combating certain types of leukemia must be weighed against the increasing incidence of the more "highly fatal" varieties.

Finally, it is becoming clear that huge new hospitals, impressive technical advances, and ever–increasing numbers of health–care professionals have done less than expected to improve our survival at either end of the life cycle. The United States still ranks 15th in the world in overall infant mortality—17th for male life expectancy at birth and eighth for female.[13]

These therapeutic shortcomings have fueled a growing dissatisfaction with the way medicine is practiced. To many patients primary care seems increasingly mechanical, perfunctory, and impersonal, medical functions specialized and fragmented. Fifteen years ago, the physician was without question the most highly respected member of society. Today, more and more questions are raised about the role and performance of doctors. Though some opinion polls continue to indicate high levels of public trust and respect, others offer a less sanguine picture; according to a recent Gallup poll, for example, a sick, angry, and mistrustful 40 percent of the public "does not feel that physicians are highly ethical and honest."

The continuous questioning of the effectiveness, safety, and cost of medical care, of the manner in which it is delivered, and of the motives and attitudes of those who deliver it has contributed to a broader reevaluation of the theoretical foundations on which modern medicine is based.

The governing perspective of medical practice which Engel describes as "biomedical,"[14] owes it conceptual power to the Cartesian vision of the body as a machine and much of its motivating force to nineteenth century scientists who discovered that certain diseases were associated with the presence of bacteria. This mechanistic and reductionistic model shaped the work of a century of investigators who sought with great success to isolate the specific bacteriological, physiological, and biochemical causes of physical and emotional illness, to discover and synthesize their pharmacological remedies.

Over the last half century, the notable achievements of this approach—the discovery, for example, of antibiotics which selectively attack offending bacteria; of exogenous insulin to replace depleted pancreatic cells; of L–dopa to provide precursors for neurotransmitters that are lacking in Parkinson's disease—have tended to obscure its inherent limitations. This model is in general unsuitable for preventng disease or promoting health: making its purveyors increasingly specialized and its recipients passive; relying on treatments which may themselves be debilitating; and neglecting the larger psychosocial and economic context in which people become sick or stay well.

In the last several years, in the wake of widespread lay and professional dissatisfaction with the costs and benefits of biomedicine, researchers and clinicians (including those represented in this volume) have begun to revise and enlarge this traditional model. They have drawn heavily on the psychosomatic tradition to which biomedicine gave birth, as well as on newer perspectives and practices derived from modern public health research studies. Many have been influenced by such newly developed technologies as biofeedback and by the recent proliferation of self–care techniques. Others have enlarged their perspectives historically and cross–culturally to include information which suggests that Western biomedicine is far less important in promoting health than changes in the economy, in agriculture, and in sanitation.[15] They have begun to adopt attitudes and techniques derived from ancient healing systems that address themselves to "balancing the whole person" rather than fighting disease.

The ground rules that follow outline a few of the perspectives of this emerging integral or holistic model. They also provide examples of the evidence—some tentative, some hard—on which these perspectives are based and some of the ways they have changed the practices of those who have adopted them.

GROUND RULES FOR INTEGRAL MEDICINE

1. *Integral practitioners recognize that distinctions between body, mind, and spirit are peculiar to the last several hundred years of Western thought and that all states of disease and health are at once physical, mental, and spiritual.* They are keenly aware that the individual's lifestyle and attitudes are crucial in producing and healing illnesses ordinary considered physical as well as the psychological ones.[16] For example, time–obsessed, hard–driving type A personalities have a far higher incidence of cardiovascular disease than more easygoing people,[17] and depressed individuals recover more slowly from illness than others.[18] Integral

practitioners know that people who experience what Viktor Frankl has called "meaning" and Paul Tillich "ultimate concern" may survive even the most overwhelming physical damage, or emotional turmoil, while those who feel despair will succumb to far smaller threats. They recognize and actively utilize faith and hope—essential parts of the placebo response—as therapeutic tools.[19]

2. *Integral practitioners understand that people are part of a network of human relations which includes their family, their community, and their society.* During the last 20 years, family therapists have demonstrated the importance of patterns of family relations in precipitating and shaping emotional disorders in individual family members. More recently, we have become aware that the physiological state of people with a variety of conditions including hypertension[20] and diabetes[21] fluctuates with changes in their relationships to significant others. Integral practitioners therefore devote much of their time and energies to working therapeutically with their patients' families, helping them to change patterns which precipitate and sustain illness.[22]

Similarly, integral practitioners—like other public–health–minded physicians—prefer to treat individuals in their social, economic, and ecological contexts. Treatment of the lead–intoxicated child with chelating agents is doomed to failure unless the child's physical surroundings change; administration of vitamins is absurd in the face of poverty which continues to make proper nutrition impossible, and it is inadequate in a society which encourages children to subsist on processed junk food.

3. *Integral practitioners are as concerned with maintaining and improving the quality of health as they are with alleviating specific illnesses.* Instead of regarding health as the absence of disease, integral practitioners encourage their clients to achieve an optimal level of physical, emotional, and social functioning. To help estimate which of their current life patterns and health practices are helpful or destructive, integral practitioners utilize a variety of self–administered questionnaires, wellness inventories, health–hazards appraisals, and life–change indices.

4. *Integral practitioners emphasize the fundamental importance of diet and exercise in maintaining health and preventing illness.* They help their clients to understand that the processed and preserved foods which form the bulk of our diet have been implicated in the production of "five of the ten leading causes of death" in the United States.[23] By encouraging their clients to reduce their intake of sugar and salt and refined, processed, and preserved foods, they assist them in adopting the kind of diet which is associated with a low incidence of chronic disease in other less "civilized" societies.[24,25]

Integral practitioners also help their clients to explore the particular type of exercise—jogging, running, aerobics, yoga, Tai Chi Chuan—which may be most helpful in preventing the diseases and disabilities which inevitably attend a sedentary lifestyle.[26,27]

5. *Integral practitioners regard their clients as active partners in diagnosis and treatment, as well as in health maintenance.* They may begin by helping them to explore the cause of their illness through words and images, reverie, and/or hypnosis. Increasingly, these explorations have confirmed what ordinary language has always revealed—that another human being may be "a pain in the neck" to a person with a stiff neck; that emotional burdens may "break people's backs"; and that loss may indeed precipitate "a broken heart."[28,29]

Having traced these so–called psychosomatic illnesses to their origins, they will encourage their clients to utilize a variety of non-invasive techniques—among them suggestion, hypnosis, biofeedback, visualization—to mobilize their own physical and mental powers to promote the healing process.[30–35] When healing is slow, they will explore the kinds of financial or emotional secondary gains that may be encouraging them to remain in the sick role. Once the illness is over, they will discuss the critical changes—in work or work habits, family relations, or recreation—that may be necessary to prevent the condition from recurring. Though they scrupulously avoid blaming clients for their illness, they do emphasize each person's individual responsibility and ability for maintaining his or her own health.

6. *Integral practitioners encourage their clients to use illness as a learning process.* People understand intuitively that they often become ill at times of stress. Sometimes individuals precipitate a physical or emotional breakdown to avoid a problem they cannot resolve or to provide themselves with a medically and socially sanctioned opportunity to withdraw and regroup their emotional forces. Integral practitioners help their clients to learn from illness. For example, the overwhelming trauma of a heart can be a lever for reevaluating the deadly pace of one's life. Even terminal cancer patients have been able to wrest an exhilarating and satisfying understanding of lifelong patterns of behavior from the illness which is killing them.[36]

7. *Integral practitioners may use diagnostic and treatment methods drawn from a variety of healing traditions.* Stimulated by accounts of the effectiveness of other health–care practices—the use of acupuncture to produce analgesia, of yogic exercises to reduce blood presssure and to slow heart rate—many integral practitioners are learning and using techniques that are fundamental to radically different systems of healing. Some have adopted as yet unproved diagnostic methods which

are based on the belief—common to many cultures—that certain parts of the body—including the ear, iris, sclera, radial pulse, the sole of the foot, the palm and the tongue—can reveal information about the health of the entire body.[37,38] Others have combined therapeutic techniques such as laying–on–of–hands,[39,40] meditation, [41,42] and acupuncture[43,44] with Western medical practices.

8. *Integral practitioners treat people, not illness.* The basic thrust of integral medicine is the restoration of what is known in the Hippocratic canon as the *Vix Medicatrix Naturae*, the healing force of nature. Instead of attempting to suppress symptoms, integral practitioners regard them as indicators of disharmony pointing to the origins of distress. Instead of trying to eradicate an illness, the integral practitioner tries to strengthen the body so that it is better able to rid itself of disease.

For example, integral practitioners are unlikely to use suppressive or palliative agents like steroids and aspirin to treat rheumatoid arthritis. Instead, they may use a variety of modalities to improve the physical and emotional well–being of the person who has rheumatoid arthritis—guided imagery techniques which may work by activating the immune system; biofeedback to reduce the stress which precipitates acute attack; nutritional counseling to alter the body's biochemical balance; hydrotherapy, exercise, and massage to mobilize limbs and joints; and family counseling to discover and resolve the patterns of relating that encourage the need for secondary gain.

9. *Integral practitioners try to create therapeutic settings which maximize the healing process.* A number of the authors in this volume emphasize the importance of the setting in which health care takes place and the need to replace large, impersonal, illness–oriented hospitals and clinics with small organizational structures which are committed to responding quickly, respectfully, and flexibly to people's individual needs. Health–care professionals in these settings encourage those who come for help to participate in shaping the kind of help they receive. In such a context, patients can easily become partners in their own treatment and, eventually, participate in the treatment of others.

10. *Integral practitioners feel they are responsible for helping to change the social and economic conditions which perpetuate ill health.* As did the great nineteenth century pathologist Virchow, many modern practitioners believe that "medicine is a social science and politics nothing but medicine on a grand scale."[45] Some may confine their efforts at change to making the principles and discoveries of integral medicine more accessible to their colleagues. Others may expand their efforts to include teaching classes in these techniques and attitudes to local schools or community groups. Others may testify against the health–

denying nutritional and pharmacological practices which pervade many of our schools, hospitals, and senior citizens' homes. Still others may participate in groups such as the Medical Committee for Human Rights or the Physicians for Social Responsibility which challenge the economic, military, and industrial practices—war and nuclear development, poverty, and industrial pollution—that seem to threaten the health of all of us.

Conclusion

The practice of integral medicine includes a scientific perspective of modern biomedicine and an emphasis on natural healing derived from the older Hippocratic tradition. It expands these with techniques derived from many cultures and tempers this amalgam with a uniquely modern emphasis on client education and self–care. It is this synthesis, not any technique which may be adapted to it, which defines integral medicine, and animates the therapeutic approaches described in this volume.

References

1. U.S. Department of Health, Education and Welfare. Cited in *Business Week*, September 4, 1978.
2. Office of Technology Assessment, U.S. Department of Health, Education and Welfare. *Assessment of new technologies of health and medical care*, 1978.
3. Knowles, J. Doing better and feeling worse, health in the United States. *Proceedings of the American Academy of Arts and Sciences. Deadalus.* Winter, 1977, *196*(1).
4. Report to the President from the President's Commission on Mental Health. Washington, D.C.: Vol. 1. Superintendent of Documents, U.S. Government Printing Office, 1978.
5. National Center for Health Statistics. *Statistics of the Bureau of Health and Vital Statistics.* February, 1968, 7(2).
6. Evans, H. E. Tonsillectomy and adenoidectomy: Review and public evidence for and against T and A. *Clinical Pediatrics.* 1968, 7(2), 71–75.
7. United States House of Representatives, Committee on Interstate and Foreign Commerce. Cost and quality of health care: Unnecessary surgery. Washington, D.C.: Superintendent of Documents, U.S. Government Printing Office, 1976.
8. Illich, I. *Medical nemesis.* New York: Bantam, 1977.

9. U.S. Department of Health, Education and Welfare. *Report of the secretary's commission on medical malpractice.* Washington, D.C., Superintendent of Documents, U.S. Government Printing Office, 1973.

10. Brecher, E. M., & the Consumer Reports editors. *Licit and illicit drugs: The consumer's union report on narcotics, stimulants, depressants, inhalants, hallucinogens and marijuana, including caffeine, nicotine and alcohol.* Boston: Little Brown, 1973.

11. Klerman, G. Mental health: Recommendations for public policy. In Carlson R. and Cunningham (Eds.), *Future directions in health care.* Cambridge, Ballinger, 1978.

12. Enstron, J. E., & Austin, D. F. Interpreting cancer survival rates. *Science,* 1977, *195,* 847–851.

13. Bureau of the Census, U.S. Department of Commerce. *Statistical Abstract of the United States.* Washington, D. C., Superintendent of Documents, U.S. Government Printing Office, 1977.

14. Engel, G. L. The need for a new medical model: A challenge for biomedicine. *Science,* 1977, *196,* 129–136.

15. Dubos, R. *Mirage of health.* New York: Harper & Row, 1959.

16. Pelletier, K. *Mind as healer, mind as slayer.* New York: Dell, 1977.

17. Rosenman, R., & Friedman, M. *Type A behavior and your heart.* New York: Knopf, 1974.

18. Imboden, J. B. Psychosocial determinants of recovery. *Advances in Psychosomatic Medicine (Vol 8.).* Basel: Darger, 1972, p. 142–155.

19. Benson, H. *The mind/body effect.* New York: Simon & Schuster, 1979.

20. Hoebel, F. C. Coronary artery disease and family interaction: A study of risk modification. In Watzlawick and Weakland (Eds.), *The interactional view,* 1976, p. 362–375.

21. Minuchin, S., Rosman, B., & Baker, L. *Psychosomatic families.* Cambridge, Ma.: Harvard, 1978.

22. Jaffe, D. This volume.

23. United States Senate Select Committee on Nutrition and Human Needs. *Dietary Goals for the United States.* Washington, D.C.: U.S. Senate, February, 1977.

24. Burkitt, D. P. The diseases of civilization. *British Medical Journal,* February 3, 1973. *1,* 1274–1278.

25. Rodale, R. This volume.

26. Ardell, D. Exercise and health. In A. Hastings, J. Fadiman, & J. Gordon (Eds.), *Holistic medicine.* Washington, D.C.: NIMH, in press.

27. Mandel, E., & Harlow, J. This volume.

28. Holmes, T., & Rahe, R. The social readjustment rating scale. *Journal of Psychosomatic Research,* 1976, *II,* 213–218.

29. Parkes, C. N., Benjamin, B., & Fitzgearald, R. G. Broken heart: A statistical study of increased mortality among widowers. *British Medical Journal,* 1969, *1,* 740–743.

30. Bresler, D. This volume.

31. Jaffe, D., & Bresler, D. This volume.

32. Shealy, C. M. This volume.

33. Simonton, O. C., & Simonton, S. This volume.

34. Miller, E. This volume.

35. Pelletier, K. This volume.

36. Simonton, O. C., & Simonton, S. *Getting well again.* New York: Tarcher, 1978.

37. Bresler, D. E., Kroenig, R. J. & Oleson, T.D. An experimental evaluation of auricular diagnosis. *Pain,* 1980, *8,* 217–229.

38. Motoyama, H. *Science and the evolution of consciousness.* Brookline, Ma.: Autumn Press, 1978.

39. Krieger, D. This volume.

40. Swearingen, R. This volume.

41. Benson, H. *The relaxation response.* New York: William Morrow, 1975.

42. Bresler, D. E. This volume.

43. Kroening, R. J., Volen, M. P., & Bresler D. E. This volume.

44. Brenner, P. This volume.

45. Rosen, G. *From medical police to social medicine.* New York: Watson, 1974.

Part II

MIND AS HEALER

In the early 1960s, Neal Miller's pioneering studies demonstrated that laboratory animals could achieve a degree of conscious control over their autonomic nervous systems. A few years later, Western scientists began to document the ability of yogis to alter profoundly a variety of bodily functions, including heart rate, temperature, and respiration. Since then, attempts to induce ordinary individuals to regulate their own internal functions—to help sufferers from psychosomatic and stress–related disease to reverse the pathologic process which afflicts them—have been increasing. Some investigators and clinicians use ancient meditative techniques to help bring about generalized states of relaxation or to control specific functions. Biofeedback technology has offered these and other practitioners and patients a way to monitor their efforts and improve their abilities. Meanwhile, techniques that were peripheral to the mainstream of medical care—such as hypnosis, visualization procedures and autogenic training—have been reexamined and recalled to clinical practice.

The essays in this section document the work of clinicians who have used these methods, singly or in combination, to help their patients to mobilize the healing powers of their minds.

In Chapter 2, Dr. David Bresler reviews the evidence implicating stress in a variety of illnesses and introduces the reader to "conditioned relaxation," a practical way for reducing stress that can be employed by health–care professionals or lay people.

David E. Bresler, Ph.D., is the founder of the Bresler Center Medical Group in West Los Angeles, California and the executive director of the Center for Integral Medicine. He is the author of numerous articles and publications related to integral medicine, including *Free Yourself From Pain* (Simon and Schuster, 1979) with Richard Trubo and *Future Medicine: Health in the 21st Century* (Simon & Schuster, 1979). Dr. Bresler was formerly an adjunct assistant professor of Anesthesiology, Gnathology and Occlusion, and Psychology, in the UCLA Schools of Medicine, Dentistry, and the College of Letters and Sciences, and the director of the Pain Control Unit of the UCLA Hospital & Clinics.

Chapter 3, by Dr. Emmett E. Miller, offers the views of a hypnotherapist on approaching stress–related illness through relaxation, suggestion, and imagery.

Dr. Miller received his medical training at Albert Einstein College of Medicine in New York and Kaiser Foundation Hospital in Oakland, California. He practiced family medicine in Carmel, California from 1970 to 1975. During this time, he pursued his studies of psychosomatic medicine, especially approaches emphasizing the training of individuals—including those with and those without apparent disease—in techniques of psychophysiological control. Among these were autogenic training, yoga, medical hypnotherapy, biofeedback, meditation, movement therapy, and cognitive behavioral therapy. From these and other Eastern and Western disciplines, he selected those techniques which proved to be objectively effective in helping individuals facilitate their healing response. These approaches and his experiences with them are presented in his two books: *Selective Awareness* (E. Miller, 1975), and *Feeling Good—How to Stay Healthy* (Prentice-Hall/Spectrum, 1978), and in a series of self–guiding cassette tapes he has produced.

Dr. Miller currently practices psychosomatic medicine and hypnotherapy in California and Oahu, subspecializing in wellness enhancement and the treatment of stress–related diseases. He also leads lay and professional classes and workshops, and performs consulting services to public and private organizations.

Dennis Jaffe and David Bresler, in Chapter 4, present a technique of guided imagery which may be used both diagnostically and therapeutically. The authors offer case material illustrating the application of their methods.

Dennis T. Jaffe, Ph.D., is co-director of the Health Studies Program at Saybrook Institute, San Francisco. He is a lecturer in the department of psychiatry of the UCLA School of Medicine. Dr. Jaffe is director of Learning for Health, a psychosomatic medicine clinic, and president-elect of the Association for Humanistic Psychology.

Dr. Jaffe is author and coauthor of several books, including *Healing from Within* (Knopf, 1980), *Abnormal Psychology in the Life Cycle* (Harper & Row, 1978), *TM: Discovering Inner Energy and Overcoming Stress* (Delacorte, 1974), *Number Nine: Autobiography of an Alternate Counseling Service* (Harper & Row, 1973), and *Worlds Apart: Young People and Drug Programs* (Vintage, 1973).

Finally, Dr. Kenneth Pelletier's Chapter 5 moves beyond individual care to survey the frontiers of biofeedback, the most widely used and carefully researched of the mental techniques for controlling physiological functioning.

Dr. Pelletier is an assistant clinical professor in the Departments of Psychiatry and Medicine at the University of California School of Medicine in San Francisco, Assistant Professor, Department of Public Health, University of California, Berkeley, California. Dr. Pelletier was a Woodrow Wilson Fellow and studied at the C. G. Jung Institute in Zurich, Switzerland. He has published over 100 professional journal articles in behavioral medicine, clinical biofeedback, and neurophysiology.

Dr. Pelletier is also coauthor of *Consciousness: East and West* (New York: Harper and Row, 1976) and author of *Mind as Healer, Mind as Slayer: A Holistic Approach to Preventing Stress Disorders* (New York: Delacorte and Delta, 1977), *Toward a Science of Consciousness* (New York, Delacorte and Delta, 1978), *Holistic Medicine: From Stress to Optimum Health* (New York: Delacorte & Delta, 1979), and *Longevity: Fulfilling Our Biological Potential* (New York, Delacorte and Delta, 1981).

Chapter 2

CONDITIONED RELAXATION

The Pause that Refreshes

David E. Bresler, Ph.D.

One of my colleagues tells the story of a man brought into an emergency room with severe third–degree burns on both ears. After immediate treatment was administered, a doctor asked the patient how he had sustained such a peculiar injury.

"Well," the man replied, "I tend to be a very nervous individual. I just can't relax. Just about everything that happens is stressful to me. Even the most trivial things make me completely fall apart. I can barely function in the modern world.

"I was home ironing this morning," he continued, "and the telephone rang. I got so nervous, flustered and confused that instead of lifting up the telephone receiver, I lifted up the iron, and burned my ear."

The doctor was startled by the unusual story. "You certainly do sound like a stressed individual," he said. "But tell me—how did you damage the *other* ear?"

Without hesitation, the patient responded, "I had to call the ambulance, didn't I?"

Humor aside, the stress of modern–day living has become a ferocious enemy of man. Health statistics in the U.S. scream out that we deal with stress very poorly. Lewis Thomas, president of the Memorial Sloan–Kettering Cancer Center, believes that relative to the universe, "we are the delicate part, transient and vulnerable as cilia."[1] Too often, we are simply unable to cope, and as a result, stress–related illness has become the major health problem in the modern world.

LIFE STRESS AND ILLNESS

For decades, researchers have suspected that there is an important link between stress and physical illness. Now, the relationship has been well–documented by hundreds of studies and thousands of individual medical histories.

Consider the three sets of identical twins studied by Dr. William A. Greene, University of Rochester psychiatrist, during the 1960s.[2] One twin from each set was a victim of leukemia. According to Greene, each of the leukemia patients had experienced a major psychological upheaval in her life immediately before the ailment manifested itself. Perhaps, concluded Greene, stress might then be considered a precipitating factor in cancer even more important than heredity.

This hypothesis has been substantiated by other researchers. Lawrence LeShan, former chief of the psychology department at the Institute of Applied Biology in New York, has studied hundreds of cancer patients over a period of a dozen years.[3–5] The majority of these individuals had endured a severe emotional trauma early in life, such as the death of a parent.

In David M. Kissen's study of 218 lung cancer patients, many of them had experienced the death or absence of a parent during childhood,[6,7] work–related problems or particularly long–term marital difficulties in adult life. These patients, said Kissen, also had "poor outlets for emotional discharge" and thus tended to manifest their pent–up emotions in a physical way.

Eugene Pendergrass, former president of the American Cancer Society, has publicly conceded that there may be a relationship between psychological stress and cancer.[8] According to Pendergrass,

> Psychological factors sometimes have a marked influence on the behavior and rate of growth of cancer once it has occurred in the human body. It is not unreasonable to postulate that this could result from the interaction of psychological factors and hormonal levels. I want to make it clear that I am not suggesting the psy-

chologic factors act as an initial causative agent in the occurrence of cancer. I am only suggesting that they sometimes have an influence of pre–existing cancer and may have an influence on susceptibility to cancer.

A link between stress and coronary artery disease is also quite clear. Dr. Flanders Dunbar at the Columbia Presbyterian Medical Center in New York noted more than three decades ago that many heart–attack victims were self–made professionals who led very trying lives.[9] According to Dunbar, they were victims of "compulsive striving" who would "would rather die than fail."

Drs. Meyer Friedman and Ray H. Roseman, in their book, *Type A Behavior and Your Heart,* conclude that people with "striving personalities" are prime candidates for heart disease, hypertension and other physical ailments.[10] These "Type A" individuals live their lives according to the calendar and the clock. They do everything rapidly— working, walking, eating. They can't do only one thing at a time, and feel guilty about "doing nothing." They are "one–man shows" who tend to do everything themselves, and they go through life with clenched fists and tightened bodies. According to Friedman and Rosenmann, over 90 percent of the males under age 60 who have heart attacks display "Type A'" behavior.

Stress is not only related to illness, it also appears to accelerate the aging process. According to pioneer stress researcher Hans Selye, "What we call aging is nothing more than the sum total of all the scars left by the stress of life." [11]

One of the most powerful stressors known is a sudden change in one's life situation. Thomas Holmes, M.D., professor of psychiatry at the University of Washington, has devised a "Schedule of Recent Experience"—a compilation of the 44 most stressful life events that appear to influence health and illness.[12–14] He assigned each "life event" a numerical rating or "scale value," ranging from 11 to 100 based upon its impact on the person.

The death of a spouse ranks highest on the scale, with a score of 100. Human beings face no more stressful event. Also ranking very high are divorce, a jail term, and personal injury or illness. Ten of the 15 top crises are related to the family in some way. Interestingly, positive changes in one's life are also stressful—such as marriage or outstanding personal achievement. Although a vacation is usually a desirable, pleasant activity, representing a change from the norm, it, too, typically involves some stress.

According to Holmes, if your total life change score is over 300 points for one year, you have almost an 80 percent chance of becoming sick in the near future. If your score falls into the 200 to 299 point range, you have about a 50 percent chance of becoming ill. A score of 150 to 199 points yields a 37 percent chance of sickness.

Research by Holmes and his associate, Richard H. Rahe, M.D., indicate that the scale is applicable regardless of race, culture, and age. In study after study, its validity has been substantiated. When Rahe evaluated the stress of 2,500 Navy men on shipboard duty, those who had recently undergone marital or family changes went on sick call 36 percent more often than those without such experiences.[15] Holmes studied the life changes of 100 college football players just before the start of the season. Based on the scores they received on the Social Readjustment Rating Scale, he classified them as either high, medium, or low risk for injuries. When the season had ended three months later, 9 percent in the low–risk group, 25 percent in the medium–risk group, and 50 percent in the high risk had been hurt.

Dr. Sidney Cobb has found that the stress of job loss and unemployment has a staggering impact upon automobile workers in Detroit.[16] Cobb, now a professor of community health and psychiatry at Brown University, studied 100 men who had been laid off from their jobs on the auto assembly lines. He began monitoring their health six weeks before the layoffs and continued doing so for a full two years. The results were startling.

According to Cobb, the unemployed workers committed suicide at a rate 30 times above the norm. Among the 100 men studied, eight cases of arthritis developed, six of severe depression, five of hypertension (which necessitated hospitalization), three of hair falling out, two of high blood pressure, and one of gout. The families of these unemployed workers also felt the impact. For example, three wives developed cases of peptic ulcers, a rare ailment for women, serious enough to require hospitalization.

THE UNSEEN ENEMY

Chronic psychosocial stress is an unfortunate companion of twentieth century humanity. True, stress has been a part of our existence since prehistoric times, but in prehistoric times, we were perfectly designed to deal with the acute or short–term stresses we faced. When a person sensed the presence of a wild animal nearby, the reaction was one of "fight or flight." That is, either the life–threatening enemy was fought off, or we fled from it.

Physiologically, the sympathetic nervous system would shift into emergency gear during moments of acute stress. The bloodstream would be inundated with adrenalin and other stress hormones. The pulse and respiration rates would quicken, and blood pressure would rise rapidly. There would be dramatic changes in the body's electrical activity, and perspiration would dampen hands and brow. Pupils would dilate, throat would tighten, and the neck and upper back would become tense. Nostrils would flare out to aid respiration. The pelvis would become rigid, numbing genitals and tightening the anus. These changes permitted immediate reaction to the crisis situation, and through either fight or flight it was usually resolved within minutes. The body would then enter a regenerative phase to prepare for future emergencies.

Modern–day individuals are faced with a far different situation. The bodies we live in were beautifully designed for survival on this planet 10,000 years ago, but in many ways they're obsolete for today's world. The major stressors we encounter are not usually resolved by the fight–or–flight response. For example, consider the fear of increasing crime rates and the concern over smog–infested skies. After all, where can most of us run in order to escape crime or increasingly polluted skies? Whom can we fight?

There are so many pressures inherent in contemporary living that very few people avoid stress–related disease. Even worse than their number is the fact that many modern–day stressors never seem to end. Our bodies are constantly activated to fight a host of invisible enemies, from inflation to the threat of nuclear holocaust. As adrenalin and other stress hormones continue to race through us, our pulse rates, respiration rates, and blood pressures remain high. Our flexor and extensor muscles are constantly tensed, and the effect is similar to what happens to your car when you step on the accelerator and brake at the same time.

Over time we slowly burn ourselves out, since our bodies rarely get a chance to relax and restore themselves. As our overloaded systems become exhausted, we tend to develop the characteristic afflictions of civilization—high blood pressure, heart disease, lung disease, ulcers, asthma, arthritis, cancer, depression, and a host of other psychophysical problems.

In short, evolution hasn't kept up with technology. We're stuck in obsolete bodies and have difficulty coping with the chronic anxieties of modern life.

What Can Be Done About It?

As a practitioner of integral medicine, I think it's important to point out that each person experiences the effects of stress in his or her own unique way. Accordingly, there are as many stress–reduction plans as there are people, and each of us must find out for ourselves what works best. Many different techniques have been recommended—including both active and passive types of relaxation. The active approaches range from jogging to swimming to yoga to dancing. Each involves muscular activity, followed by profound muscle relaxation, and a sense of well–being. Active relaxing can also occur on a psychological level, in the form of an activity such as reading.

Passive relaxation techniques include massage and manipulation, which directly relax the muscles and, in the process, relax the mind as well. The mind and the body can also be rested by using a variety of psychological approaches. One of the best known of these techniques is Transcendental Meditation, or TM, first introduced in the United States by Maharishi Mahesh Yogi in 1959. The technique, which can be learned in just a few hours, involves sitting comfortably in a chair with your eyes closed, and then silently repeating a "mantra" (a specific but meaningless sound) over and over for 20 minutes.

In studies by Robert Keith Wallace and Herbert Benson, M.D., TM was found to cause declines in heart rate, respiratory rate, cardiac output, oxygen consumption, and carbon dioxide elimination.[17] Simultaneously, there was a rise in skin resistance, indicating a reduction of stress.

Wallace found that people who regularly practiced TM simply felt healthier. In a survey of 394 meditators, 67 percent said that their physical health had improved, and 84 percent reported an improvement in their mental well–being.

Another effective approach to relaxation is autogenic training, a system developed more than 40 years ago by German psychiatrist Johannes H. Schultz.[18] This technique is used to induce various positive physical states by passive concentration on specific commands ("My heartbeat is calm and regular," or "My right arm is heavy"). Silently repeating these phrases over and over tends to induce extremely deep states of relaxation.

It seems obvious to me that these and other stress management techniques can significantly reduce the afflictions of civilization, for they provide an easy and effective way to end the long–term fight–or–flight response which now works against us. Many stress researchers believe that appropriate stress management can help cut cholesterol levels and the incidence of high blood pressure and heart attacks. Relaxation techniques also provide a positive alternative to smoking (which is a major health hazard) and to excessive drinking, drug taking, and overeating, as such forms of consumption are said to contribute significantly to many health problems.

Although many doctors advise their chronically ill patients to relax, few bother to teach them *how* to do it. Given what is known about the harmful effects of excessive stress, it seems amazing to me that Americans are not systematically taught how to relax. Neither my parents nor my friends ever taught me. I went to school for a long time, and none of my teachers ever taught me. Nor did any of my doctors.

A relaxation exercise is so basic and yet so simple that it might best be introduced into the public schools in the first grade. This could be a significant way of preventing the unnecessary suffering of patients with stress-related disorders reducing, as well, the staggering costs of modern medical care.

Why Conditioned Relaxation?

My own relaxation system—called "Conditioned Relaxation"—emerged from my experiences at UCLA as a method particularly effective for dealing with pain. Unlike TM, it does not require a mantra. Once mastered—through diligent practice—a state of relaxation can be achieved almost instantaneously by taking a single "signal breath."

Conditioned Relaxation is based on the work of Ivan Pavlov,[19] the Russian psychophysiologist, whose experiments with dogs first demonstrated the conditioning process. Pavlov rang a bell, showed a hungry dog some meat, and —of course—the animal salivated. After repeating this procedure many times, Pavlov eliminated the middle step—that is, he rang the bell but did not show the meat to the dog. Because of the repeated pairing of the bell and the meat, the dog had become conditioned to salivate whenever he heard the bell.

Conditioning is the most fundamental form of learning on the planet. Most sophisticated life forms—from worms to guinea pigs to cats to dogs—learn this way. When your cat—or even your goldfish—sees you approaching at feeding time, he will usually become highly excited, even before seeing the food. Our primitive nervous system learns this way as well.

In Conditioned Relaxation, these same principles of classical conditioning are applied to allow you to relax on command—even when you're unable to go through an entire relaxation exercise. Just as the bell became an automatic signal for Pavlov's dog to salivate, a "signal breath" can be used to help your body relax instantaneously.

There are enormous benefits in learning to relax on command. For example, if you begin to experience excessive stress while driving on the freeway, you would obviously be unable to perform most relaxation techniques. But it would certainly be possible to take a quick signal breath that would immediately induce relaxation.

Everyone can learn Conditioned Relaxation and benefit from it. No unusual mental capabilities are necessary, and nor any particular educational experiences. The only requirements are patience and practice. Relaxation cannot be forced. Although you can voluntarily tighten or tense many of your muscles, you can't voluntarily relax them. You can only *allow* them to relax by not contracting them. By analogy, try forcing yourself to urinate, to remember a name, or to go to sleep. You can't make these happen. In the same way, you can't make yourself relax; you can only *allow* it to occur.

Some people reap the benefits of Conditioned Relaxation the first or second time they try it. Others need to practice it patiently and persistently until positive benefits are achieved. Just as in hitting a tennis ball, your muscles must learn to perform in a particular way, once you've developed the necessary skills through diligent practice, you don't need to work nearly as hard to keep them performing optimally.

THE BREATH OF LIFE

Breathing is literally the way of life, for the air around us is a vital source of nourishment. Each time we breathe, we draw oxygen into the body's cells and tissues, where it is used in the burning of the body's fuel and the production of energy.

According to the philosophy of yoga, breathing controls the flow of prana—the cosmic life force—into the body. The nose, it is believed, is the proper instrument for breathing, rather than the mouth. If you pay close attention to your breathing, you'll notice that it varies according to your moods. You breath differently, for example, when you're happy as opposed to sad, bored as opposed to excited, or calm as opposed to angry. Proper breathing can actually help to control destructive emotions, including anger, hatred, jealousy, grief, and frustration. Simply by slowing down the rhythm of breathing, which in turn reduces the heart rate, you can often eliminate tension, nervousness, or even shyness.

Compare your own breathing to that of a baby. Most likely, your breathing is centered in your upper chest, and only the thorax is involved in taking short, shallow breaths. Infants, however, instinctively know how to breathe properly. They contract their diaphragm with each inhalation, then relax it, contracting their abdominal muscles as they exhale. Try it and you'll find that this type of deep, abdominal breathing is highly relaxing.

Take a few moments now to begin working with your breathing. Sit upright in a comfortable chair, and begin breathing slowing and deeply from the abdomen. Let your breathing become very rhythmic, as each inhalation equals each exhalation in length. You may find it helpful to count as you breathe, so as you inhale, count "one thousand, two thousand, three thousand . . ." Allow each breath to be natural, flowing deep into your abdomen and flowing out on its own. Adjust your rate of breathing until your body finds its own smooth, regular, and natural rhythm.

This type of breathing is an essential prerequisite for mastering Conditioned Relaxation, so before you proceed further spend some time working on your breathing until you feel that you have mastered the ability to breathe slowly, deeply, and easily from the abdomen.

Preparation: Learning to Breathe

Each time you practice Conditioned Relaxation, find a quiet spot in which to do it. Don't allow yourself to be interrupted before you've completed the exercise. Take the phone off the hook and ask the children to play in another part of the house. I often park my car at the beach on my way to UCLA and perform the relaxation technique there. It's about the only place I've found where I am virtually guaranteed that I won't be distracted for several minutes.

Get yourself as comfortable as you can before beginning the exercise. Unfasten your belt, untie your shoes, loosen your tie, and remove any jewelry you may be wearing.

I recommend that you perform this exercise in a seated position, unless it is very uncomfortable for you to do so. If you lie down, you'll find that you may fall asleep before the exercise is completed. Later on you can use this exercise to help induce sleep, at which time the reclining position is obviously preferable. However, you can't learn the full technique if you fall asleep so, while practicing, a comfortable seated position is recommended.

Whereas Transcendental Meditation uses a mantra to quiet the mind, Conditioned Relaxation uses your own breathing. At the onset of the exercise, you will concentrate on your breathing as a means of keeping your mind from wandering to any stressful thoughts. At various other times throughout the exercise, you will refocus on the simple and natural act of inhaling and exhaling.

Keep in mind that there are two ways to breathe: from your chest, and from your abdomen. For this exercise, try to breathe only from your abdomen, meaning that your stomach will move in and out with each breath you take. Allow your breathing to become slow and rhythmic.

The text of the relaxation exercise is printed below. If you like, you can read it through several times and then try it. However, I would suggest that you have a friend read it to you as you perform it. Or, because most people find it difficult to arrange for another person to read the exercise to them two or three times a day, I strongly recommend that you read the text into a cassette tape recorder and then perform the exercise while the tape is being played back.

It's advisable initially to work with a friend or a tape recorder for two reasons: first of all, it is difficult to remember the entire exercise, and secondly, it's often hard to pace yourself properly. If you learn the exercise the wrong way, you'll only be hurting yourself. A friend or the tape recorder can serve as an important guide to keep you on the proper track.

If you (or your friend) are a fast reader, now is the time to slow down. As you read the following text into the microphone of your tape recorder, do it slowly and deliberately. Let each thought penetrate deep into your mind before you begin the next one. As a general rule, speak slowly, pause about three seconds each time there is an ellipsis (. . .), and about six seconds between paragraphs.

Now, let's get started.

CONDITIONED RELAXATION*

This tape contains a Conditioned Relaxation exercise which you can use any time you wish to reach a deep state of gentle relaxation.

Before beginning, take a moment to get comfortable and relax . . . Sit upright in a comfortable chair and loosen any tight clothing or jewelry or shoes that might distract you. Make sure you won't be interrupted for a few minutes . . . Take the telephone off the hook

---

* © 1975 by David E. Bresler, Ph.D

if necessary . . . Now take a few slow, deep abdominal breaths . . . Inhale . . . Exhale . . . Inhale . . . Exhale.

Focus your attention on your breathing throughout this exercise and recognize how easily slow deep breathing alone can help to produce relaxation. Let your body breathe itself, according to its own natural rhythm . . . Slowly and deeply.

Now let's begin the exercise with what we call a "signal breath," a special message that tells the body we are ready to enter a state of deep relaxation. The signal breath is taken as follows . . . Exhale . . . Take a deep breath in through your nose . . . Then blow it out through your mouth.

You may notice a kind of "tingling"sensation when you take the signal breath. Whatever you feel is a signal or message to your body that will become associated with relaxation as you practice this exercise over and over again. Soon, simply taking the signal breath will produce the same degree of relaxation that you'll get by completing the entire exercise.

Breathe slowly and deeply . . . As you concentrate your attention on your breathing, focus your eyes on an imaginary spot in the center of your forehead . . . Look at the spot as if you are trying to see it from the inside of your head . . . Raise your eyes up so as to stare at that spot from the inside of your head. Concentrate your attention on it . . . The more you are able to concentrate on the spot, the better your relaxation response will be.

As you continue to focus attention on the spot, you might notice that your eyelids have beome quite tense . . . That's fine, for we want to teach your body the difference between tension and relaxation. Your eyelids, controlled by some very small muscles in your body, become easily tired and fatigued as they become more and more tense. When I count to three, we'll demonstrate the difference between tension and relaxation by allowing your eyelids to gently close, allowing feelings of tension to quickly melt away.

One . . . Two . . . Three . . . Close your eyelids firmly but not tightly, and as they close, sense the soothing feeling of relaxation radiating around your eyes . . . the top of your eyes . . . the bottom . . . the sides . . . the front and back.

Breathe slowly and deeply . . . Feel the relaxation in your eyes, and how nice it feels . . . Let these feelings of gentle relaxation radiate all around your eyes and out to your forehead . . . to your scalp . . . around the back of your head . . . to your ears and temples . . . to your cheeks and nose . . . to your mouth and chin . . . and around to your jaw . . . As you feel all the tension flow out of your face and the area around your mouth, relax your jaw muscles . . . And as you do so, let your jaw gently open slightly so that all the tension can smoothly flow away.

Remember your breathing, slowly and deeply . . . Relax the muscles in your neck, and as you relax the back of your neck, let your head tip gently forward until your chin just about touches your chest . . . As you do so, feel all the tension flow away from the muscles in the back of your neck . . . Let this warm, gentle feeling of relaxation now radiate down into your shoulders . . . Feel the heaviness of your shoulders on your trunk as the shoulder muscles gently relax . . . This is one of the most important areas of the body to relax since we store a lot of tension in our neck and shoulders . . . Feel all the tension flow away, and sense the warm, gentle feeling of deep relaxation.

Remember your breathing, slowly and deeply . . . Let this feeling of relaxation now radiate down your arms . . . to your elbows . . . forearms . . . wrists . . . and hands . . . Spend a moment to relax each of your fingers . . . your thumb, index finger, middle finger, ring finger, little finger . . . As your hands and arms completely and gently relax, you may notice feelings of warmth and heaviness . . . Some people report pulsations or tingly sensations . . . Some can even sense their heartbeat in their fingertips . . . Others report even magnetic or pulling sensations . . . Whatever you experience is your body's way of expressing relaxation . . . Remember, you cannot force yourself to relax, you can only allow yourself to relax . . . Trust your body . . . It knows what to do.

Remember your breathing, slowly and deeply . . . Relax your chest . . . and abdomen . . . and let this feeling of relaxation radiate around your sides and ribs, as waves of relaxation cross your shoulder blades to meet at your upper back . . . middle back . . . and lower back . . . Feel all the muscles on either side of your spine softly relax . . . Let your spine carry the weight of your trunk as your back muscles relax more and more deeply . . . Let this feeling of gentle relaxation now radiate down into your pelvic area . . . to your buttocks . . . sphincter muscle . . . genitals . . . Feel your whole pelvic area open up and gently relax . . . Relax your thighs . . . knees . . . calves . . . ankles . . . and feet . . . Spend a moment to relax each toe. . . your big toe, second toe, third toe, fourth toe, and little toe . . . Breathe slowly and deeply . . . Relax and enjoy it.

Now that your body is gently relaxed and quiet, take a moment, starting from the top of your head working down, to lightly check to see how much relaxation you have obtained.

If there is any part of your body that is not yet fully relaxed and quiet, take a moment, starting from the top of your head working down, to lightly check to see how much relaxation you have obtained.

If there is any part of your body that is not yet fully relaxed and comfortable, simply inhale a deep breath and send it into that area, bringing soothing, relaxing, nourishing, healing oxygen into every cell of that area, comforting and relaxing it . . . As you exhale, imagine blowing out, right through your skin, any tension, tightness, pain, or discomfort in that area. Again, as you inhale, bring relaxing, healing oxygen into every cell of that area, and as you exhale, blow away, right through the skin, any tension or discomfort.

In this way you can send your breath to relax any part of your body which is not yet as fully relaxed and comfortable as it can be . . . Breathe slowly and deeply, and with each breath, allow yourself to become twice as relaxed as you were before . . . Inhale . . . Exhale . . . Twice as relaxed . . . Inhale . . . Exhale . . . Twice as relaxed.

When you find yourself quiet and fully relaxed, take a moment to enjoy it . . . Sense the gentle warmth and feeling of well–being all through your body . . . If any extraneous thoughts try to interfere, simply allow them to pass through and out of you . . . Ignore them and go back to your breathing, slowly and deeply . . . Slowly and deeply . . . Enjoy this nice state of gentle relaxation.

Now, as you concentrate on your breathing, paint a picture in your head of how you want to be . . . See yourself or any part of your body as you want it to be . . . Freely use your imagination. See the possibilities of being exactly as you want to be . . . See more clearly this vision in the center of your mind's eye.

Breathe slowly and deeply . . . Remember your wish, what you want for life . . . Strengthen it . . . Tell yourself that "every day, in every way, I feel better and better" . . . "Every day, in every way, I feel better and better" . . . "Every day in every way, my wish grows stronger and stronger" . . . "Every day, in every way, my wish grows stronger and stronger" . . . Add any other suggestions you want to make to yourself.

Remember your breathing, slowly and deeply . . . When you end this exercise, you may be surprised to notice that you feel not only relaxed and comfortable, but energized with such a powerful sense of well–being that you will easily be able to meet any demands that arise . . . To end the exercise, tell yourself that you can reach this nice gentle state of Conditioned Relaxation any time you wish by simply taking the signal breath . . . Reinforce that signal breath by concluding the exercise with it. . . . Exhale . . . Inhale deeply through your nose . . . Blow out through the mouth . . . And be well.

The Art of Diligent Practicing

If your initial experiences with Conditioned Relaxation are positive, you may be convinced that nothing will ever keep you from practicing it at least two times a day. But despite the best of intentions, be prepared for those difficult times when setting aside ten minutes for the exercise will seem like the most impossible task you've ever faced.

Here's a typical scenario that you should be prepared for: You oversleep one morning, you race in and out of the shower, dress quickly, fix yourself a fast breakfast, separate the kids who are already fighting, curse the paperboy for throwing the *Times* on the roof again, call the repairman about a malfunction in the hot water heater, and grab your shovel to dig your car out of the three–foot snowstorm that struck the previous night. Now—honestly—on a day like that, are you going to find ten minutes to practice Conditioned Relaxation?

Probably not. And that's very unfortunate, since the stress of such a morning makes the relaxation exercise all the more necessary and beneficial. I urge you to force yourself to practice the relaxation exercise twice a day, even if only in an abbreviated fashion. Although it may seem inconvenient, you will never regret doing it. The exercise should never be thought of as a chore, but rather as precious time devoted to improving your life. Nothing is more important than your health and well–being, so why not give yourself this valuable gift twice each day?

I'm reminded of the young man who once asked James Fadiman if he meditates, to which Fadiman replied, "Yes, for three minutes every day." The man laughed, expressing his doubts that any positive benefit could be obtained from only three minutes of meditation. But Fadiman responded, "I find it much better to relax for three minutes than to *not* relax for half an hour."

Some of my patients have told me they practice the Conditioned Relaxation exercise ony when their discomfort flares up. But under such circumstances, it's not unlike the leaking roof syndrome. When it's raining outside, it can't be repaired, yet when it's not raining, there's no need to fix it. If practiced only randomly, the relaxation exercise may be ineffective when it's really needed.

In order for the signal breath to become a conditioned stimulus that will reliably produce relaxation, the exercise must be practiced on a regular basis. If you stop practicing, the conditioned response will gradually fade away, but with continued practice, it will stay indefinitely.

You may be so skeptical that you don't give the exercise a chance to work. Understandably, the patient orientation for years has centered around pills and injections, conditioning us to reject such a simple, uncomplicated procedure. As the reasoning goes, "If strong medication doesn't help me, how can a few deep breaths and a relaxed limb or two do any good?"

Give this relaxation technique a fair trial and then decide whether or not it is truly beneficial. If made as much a part of the daily routine as eating and brushing teeth, it will become a positive habit rather than an intrusion on other activities.

PROBLEM SOLVING

Although Conditioned Relaxation can be learned by almost anyone motivated enough to practice it, some people do meet problems along their road to relaxation. Let me mention some of the most common difficulties encountered in learning the technique and how best to cope with them:

1. Many people find it extremely difficult to concentrate solely on the exercise itself. In such cases, the key is to stick with it. If you practice and keep practicing the exercise, you'll find that it becomes progressively easier and more effective.

2. The mind is like a child. It has grown accustomed to receiving all of your attention, and it may throw it's own kind of temper tantrum when you try to quiet it for a few moments. Even when you make every effort to concentrate on your breathing, your mind may wander without warning, distracting you in any way possible in order to reclaim your attention. For instance, in the middle of the exercise, your mind may interrupt you with thoughts like these:

> I forgot to unplug the toaster downstairs in the kitchen. And right now the toaster plug is waving in the breeze that's blowing through the window . . . Oh, no, the plug is frayed, and sparks are shooting out. They've set the cord on fire . . . The fire is spreading to the drapes . . . The drapes are burning now . . . The fire has now spread to the kitchen cabinets . . . If I get up right now and run downstairs, I can probably throw enough water on the fire to put it out. But if I keep doing this nonsensical exercise . . . Oh, no, the fire has now spread to the walls . . .

This entire monologue occurs in a flash. And it's an example of what your mind will do to try to bring you out of the exercise. Although you don't consciously or deliberately make thoughts enter your mind, you may suddenly become aware that your mind has successfully kidnapped your attention and that you are lost in thought.

The best way to deal with this situation is just to let your thoughts pass through you, as if you are invisible. Don't identify with them. Experience them as butterflies flittering around, then see them fly away, leaving you quietly behind. Don't get angry, frustrated, guilty, or worried. Don't resist them, fight them, or try to stop them. Any response you make will take you out of the relaxation experience. So instead, just go back to your breathing, without interacting with your thoughts.

Also, don't worry about forgetting something important that comes to mind while doing the exercise. Simply tell yourself that this isn't the time to think about it, and return to your breathing. You'll remember it when you finish the exercise. It will not be lost forever, no matter how hard your mind may try to convince you of that.

After you have been doing the relaxation exercise for quite some time, your mind may change its tactics. In my case, my mind has learned that the best way to distract me is with its sense of humor. On one occasion, I was flowing through the exercise very smoothly, when suddenly my mind flashed: "I forgot to get the air in my car tires changed!" It was such an outlandish thought that I could not keep from laughing, which took me right out of the relaxation experience. But I soon regained my composure, returned my concentration to my breathing, and let the thoughts pass. Just as a child gradually learns rules of behavior, so does the mind learn to be still. As you continue to practice, such distractions will become significantly less frequent.

3. Some people simply don't know what it feels like to relax. They may never have really relaxed in their lives. As a friend once said, telling a tense, nervous person to relax is like telling him to stop breathing. He simply can't do it.

For people such as this, I often recommend a few sessions of biofeedback. It helps provide them with instantaneous information as to when their various muscles are relaxing and what it feels like when they do. Biofeedback can open up the doors of perception, allowing you to taste what relaxation really is. Once it's learned, then Conditioned Relaxation can be used to its fullest potential.

4. People who don't use a tape recorder as a guide often race through the exercise and thus reap little if any benefit from it. If you don't have a tape recorder, buy an inexpensive cassette recorder so you can make your own tape or purchase a prerecorded copy. Eventually, as you become more familiar with the exercise, begin to practice

once a day with the tape and once without it to gradually become accustomed to performing the exercise on your own.

CHARTING YOUR PROGRESS

In my opinion, Conditioned Relaxation (or some suitable alternative) should be practiced at least twice daily. A useful way of keeping track of your progress is to keep a daily log.

Before each practice session, rate your subjective levels of tension or relaxation using a -10 to $+10$ scale. Thus, if you feel slightly tense, rate it -1. If you're as tense as you have ever been, rate it -10. Anything in between should be so rated. In the same way, use a $+1$ to $+10$ scale for relaxation. So if you feel slightly relaxed, rate it $+1$ and if you are totally and completely relaxed, rate it $+10$. Again, rate anything in between accordingly and enter these "before" values in your log.

After completing the relaxation exercise, rate your subjective levels of tension/relaxation again, and note these "after" values, along with any feelings of importance in your log. Once a week, calculate the algebraic sums of the daily "before"and "after" values and plot them on a progress graph to illustrate the dramatic effects of your efforts. Once you begin showing steady improvement, this will be an important incentive to help you to keep practicing your relaxation exercise diligently and regularly.

In follow–up reports from pain patients who have practiced Conditioned Relaxation for at least several weeks, the results have often been astounding. Pain relief has been the general rule rather than the exception. Many patients have learned to reduce or even stop spasticity in their muscles. Others have used the exercise to help them sleep at night. Still others report an enormous sense of well–being and rekindled feelings of self–confidence.

So why not give Conditioned Relaxation a try? Perhaps you, too, will learn to make the signal breath the pause that refreshes.

REFERENCES

1. Thomas, L. *Lives of a cell.* New York: Viking Press, 1974.
2. Green, W.A. The psychosocial setting of the development of leukemia and lymphoma. In E. M. Meyer & H. Hutchins (Eds.), *Psychophysiological aspects of cancer.* New York: New York Academy of Sciences, 1966, pp. 794–801.

3.   LeShan L. Psychological states as factors in the development of malignant disease. A critical review. *National Cancer Institute Journal*, 1959, *22*,1–18.

4.   LeShan L. A basic psychological orientation apparently associated with malignant disease. *The Psychiatric Quarterly*, 1961, *36*,314–330.

5.   LeShan, L. An emotional life–history pattern associated with neoplastic disease. *Annals of the New York Academy of Science*, 1966, *125*,780–793.

6.   Kissen, D.M. The significance of personality in lung cancer in men. In E.M. Meyer & H. Hutchins (Eds.), *Psychophysiological aspects of cancer*. New York: New York Academy of Sciences, 1966, pp. 933–945.

7.   Kissen, D.M. Psychosocial factors, personality and lung cancer in men aged 55–64. *British Journal of Medical Psychology*, 1967, *40*,29.

8.   Pendergass, E. Presidential Address to the American Cancer Society, 1959.

9.   Dunbar, F. *Emotions and bodily changes*. New York: Columbia University Press, 1947.

10. Friedman, M., & Rosenman, R.H. *Type A behavior and your heart*. New York: Alfred A. Knopf, Inc., 1974.

11. Selye, H. *Stress without distress*. Philadelphia: J.B. Lippincott Company, 1974.

12. Holmes, T.H., & Masuda, M. Life change and illness susceptibility. In: B.S. Dohrenwend & D.P. Dohrenwend (Eds.), *Stressful life events*. New York: John Wiley & Sons, 1974, pp. 45–72.

13. Holmes, T.H. *The schedule of recent experience* (SRE) published by the author, Department of Psychiatry, University of Washington, School of Medicine. 1967.

14. Holmes, T.H., & Rahe, R.H. The social readjustment rating scale. *Journal of Psychosomatic Research*, 1967, *11*,213–218.

15. Rahe, R.H. Life–change measurement as a predictor of illness. *Proceedings of the Royal Society of Medicine*, 1973, *61*,1124–1126.

16. Fier, B. Recession is causing dire illness. *Moneysworth*, June 23, 1975.

17. Wallace, R.K., & Benson, H. The physiology of meditation. *Scientific American*, February 1972, pp. 84–90.

18. Schultz, J.H., & Luthe, W. *Autogenic therapy*. New York: Grune & Stratton, Inc., 1969.

19. Pavlov, I. *Conditioned reflexes: An investigation of the physiological activity of the cerebral cortex*. New York: Oxford University Press, 1927.

Chapter 3

MIND–BODY HARMONY THROUGH DEEP RELAXATION, IMAGERY, AND AGE REGRESSION

Emmet E. Miller, M.D.

My approach to age regression therapy was developed in the course of clinical practice in general medicine, psychsomatic medicine, and hypnotherapy. Combining the features of such approaches as autogenic training, meditation, and insight therapy, it is especially useful in stress–related disorders and those associated with physical, emotional, and behavioral symptomatology.

During the last few years, in both psychotherapy and medicine, there have been major changes in approaches to the mind, the body, and the interaction between them. The popularity of Gestalt psychology, autogenic techniques, biofeedback–aided control of the "involuntary" nervous system, behavioral therapy, and hypnosis is steadily increasing. Increasingly, physicians, dentists, psychologists, and psychiatrists are incorporating hypnotherapy into their practices. Since its proven efficacy in the treatment of battlefield neurosis following World War II, hypnosis has become a familiar psychiatric tool, receiving in 1958, formal recognition by the American Medical Association. Surgeons using hypnosis note a remarkably increased speed of recovery and freedom from infection when a preoperative hypnotic induction has been performed. Self–hypnosis, learned from a competent clinician, has helped many people change their self–image and eliminate undesirable habits. Many persons feel comfortable flying in airplanes, speaking in front of the PTA meetings, or swimming in the ocean as a direct result of hypnotherapy.

DISCOVERING A NEW TOOL

My introduction to hypnosis came several years after graduation from medical school. During a social gathering, a doctor mentioned that he had used hypnosis in the treatment of a mutual friends's back pain. My eyebrows must have flown up in surprise. Medical hypnosis? I had just finished my studies at one of the country's best medical schools and not once had hypnotherapy been mentioned. I had been warned that sometimes general practitioners located far from university centers practiced certain "dubious" forms of medicine. I lowered my eyebrows soberly and gave my colleague my most skeptical look. Then I asked, "Where can I learn about this hyponosis business?"

Within the next few hours, I was seated in front of my tape recorder listening (in the most critical manner I could muster) to the tape he had loaned me. On it, Dave Elman, a lay hypnotist, was teaching a group of physicians and dentists how to incorporate hypnosis in their work. It was their first lesson, and from the questions they asked, they were as skeptical as I. After some introductory comments, he asked for a volunteer, and, following a brief induction, one of the doctors was given the suggestion that his lower jaw would become as numb as if he had just had an injection of novocaine. Mr. Elman then called up one of the dentists to test the anesthesia with a dental probe. After a few moments he blurted out, "Why, I'm scraping the periostium!" His voice showed great surprise, since this usually painful procedure brought forth no response from the subject. "What are you feeling?" asked the hypnotist. "Just a little pressure" replied the subject, who was also a bit surprised.

The amazed comments of the other doctors in the group convinced me that they were really seeing something happen. As I listened to hour after hour of instructions and demonstrations on the tape, I found I was undergoing a profound change in my thinking. Memories of pain echoed through my mind: women screaming for hours in the labor and delivery rooms, postoperative patients and cancer victims who required round the clock narcotics for freedom from agony, young and old alike who would rather have their teeth rot than spend a few hours in the dentist's chair. And here was a simply applied tech-

nique that showed promise of being of great value for relieving pain—
without the unpleasant side effects of drugs.

At this time I was working in an emergency room, which turned
out to be an excellent proving ground, when a problem initially arose.
It was easy enough to tell someone with a lacerated hand that I was
going to inject some medicine to numb the area before suturing it,
but could I risk the embarrassment of failing after proclaiming that
I could deaden the area with hypnosis? I feared my patient might
consider me odd for even suggesting such a thing. I thought about
how I had felt a few weeks earlier when I had first heard about it.

So I studied alone for weeks and practiced inducing glove anesthesia with friends, trying to summon the courage to use it in actual
clinical practice. At last the moment of truth arrived.

Late one night, a seven–year–old girl was brought to the emergency department with a laceration of the left upper eyelid. Sutures
would be needed to close the wound, but she was so scared I knew
that she would never let me come near her eye with the anesthetic
needle. Even by tying her down (a primitive procedure often used in
such cases), we would never be able to keep her eyes still enough for
the delicate procedure necessary to prevent permanent scarring, not
to mention the emotional consequences. I had two possible choices:
the rather unpleasant alternative of using powerful anesthetic agents
to put her to sleep (with all its side effects and possible complications),
or trust Dave Elman's statement on the tape that "children make the
best subjects of all."

I felt that I was really risking very little with this girl. If hypnoanesthesia failed, I could always call the anesthesiologist. I wouldn't
be too embarrassed if I failed in front of this child, and if I avoided
using the word "hypnosis" she would not be able to explain my failure
to her parents, who were in the waiting room. In my most authoritative
tone of voice, I turned to the nurse and said, "Please draw the curtains,
Miss Bennett, I'm going to use hypnoanesthesia," and set to work.

"Okay. Barbara, would you like to do this the easy way or the
hard way?" Children seldom have trouble with such questions.

"The easy way!"

"Great. Now you must do exactly as I tell you. Close your eyes
and pretend you can't open them . . . Good . . . What's your favorite
TV program?"

Any parent whose child has begged for that toy he saw on television will attest to the remarkable ease with which television programs
render a child hypersuggestible. Studies indicate that the television
watcher is in a very receptive state, one similar to, or identical with,

hypnosis. This holds true even if the television is an imaginary one. I proceeded to repeat the children's induction that I had heard on the tape and practiced so often in the privacy of my room. The smile on her face as she watched "The Beverly Hillbillies" and the tiny fluttering movements of her eyelids told me the time had come.

Gingerly, I passed the needle through one flap of skin. The lack of any movement encouraged me and I passed it through the other side and pulled the suture thread through. She was still smiling and felt nothing.

Suddenly the silence around me was broken by what sounded like ten people exhaling simultaneously. I turned, and to my surprise the entire staff of the emergency room, alerted by the nurse to the strange goings–on, had silently slipped inside the curtain. They had all been holding their breaths in anticipation of the inevitable scream of pain and were now standing in wide–eyed amazement. The suspense was over. I had passed my test. I finished the job and carried her smiling to her parents. A new day had dawned.

For the next six months, I used my new skill with increasing confidence. I used the technique in many of the cases in which I would ordinarily have used a chemical anesthetic. In addition, I found that if told to do so in this state, a patient could diminish or even halt bleeding, making minor surgery easier. Healing time was speeded up, scars were reduced in size, and pain and infection during the recovery and healing period were dramatically reduced.

But for me, this was only a beginning. Soon I found myself thinking, "If the increased relaxation and focused concentration of hypnosis could be used to eliminate pain, perhaps these techniques could be applied with equal success in other areas." Pain is one of the most dominating sensations we can experience. A person with severe pain will be unable to get up to get a cigarette, a glass of alcohol, or extra candy no matter how bad his habit is. Regardless of how angry, depressed, or frightened a person is, he will quickly forget his emotion, at least for a while, if he accidently steps on a nail. If a pain could block these problems and habits, and hypnosis could handle pain, I reasoned that hypnosis might be used to temporarily inhibit the perception of other maladaptive emotions and sensations. Perhaps temporary freedom from these compulsive emotions could help free the habits and physical symptoms they cause. Then a person could focus on the process at the root of the problems and by changing it, eliminate the symptom and free the bound emotional energy.

Age regression was the tool I used in investigating this hypothesis. It has long been known that even during the lightest states of hypnosis there is a remarkably enhanced ability to relive events that occurred in the past and to reexperience the original emotion as well. Most of us were not born with problems such as recurring depressions, cigarette habits, and headaches, so we must have learned them somewhere along the way. They are like computer programs that we have learned without our realizing it. I hoped that perhaps these unwanted programs could be traced to their source. Here the patient could be desensitized to the maladaptive emotions (e.g. fear, guilt, anger) experienced in these sensitizing events, even as my patients had been able to temporarily sensitize themselves to pain. Deprived of the driving motivation, perhaps the "program" and its resultant habit pattern would vanish. What's more, since the actual cause had been removed, there would be no tendency for recurrence or for substitution of other symptoms. Gradually the concept of Selective Awareness exploration evolved.

THE SELECTIVE AWARENESS EXPLORATION

Generally speaking, a patient or client will present a symptom. This may be a physical symptom such as a headache, an unwanted habit such as smoking, or an emotional reaction such as recurrent fear, anxiety, or anger that is experienced as maladaptive. Generally, any pattern in the individual's life which he or she can identify and label "maladaptive" can serve as a starting point for an exploration. Usually the pattern can be determined rather quickly, with only a brief history taken—how long, how severe, previous treatment, etc. At this time we can also determine whether or not there is a possibility of the symptom representing an organic problem. It should be made clear to the subject that although an exploration can be effective in helping to resolve the psychological aspects of a psychosomatic problem, medical or surgical intervention may also be desirable. One is not a substitute for the other.

After a brief explanation of what will occur, the subject is now induced to relax. States of deep relaxation and hypnosis seem to allow for much greater ability to recall memories and to alter ingrained patterns. Generally, to facilitate entrance into a receptive state, I use a highly permissive relaxation induction similar to those found in many clinical hypnosis texts and audio cassettes.

Once an adequate state of relaxation has been reached, the therapist suggests that the person drift back in time. The actual wording may go something like this:

A little while ago, before you became as relaxed as you are now,
we were talking about a problem that you have had with headaches
in the past. We talked about the possibility that those headaches
may have come on following periods of tension. As I talk to you
now, imagine that you are beginning to drift back into the past.
Imagine that you are in a time machine and are drifting back
several days, or perhaps weeks, to some fairly recent time just a
few moments before your body began to develop the tension that
caused a headache to develop. (Pause.) As this scene comes in,
you will feel very relaxed because you will go to the very beginning
of the scene. When you can make out where you are and what
you are doing, then take a deep breath in, and as you let that
breath out, tell me where you are.

Memories are "remembered" by some people, "recalled," "relived," or "reexperienced" by others, whereas other subjects simply
have vague recollections. The more analytic the subject is, the more
likely we are to get whatever the individual comes up with as a memory.
Once the memory is readily accepted, the person will relax, stop questioning, feel encouraged, and find it easier to go back to his next
memory.

The subject now describes the scene to the therapist as it unfolds,
just as though he or she has never been there before. The therapist
must be very watchful for the exact point in the memory at which
time the subject begins to show tension, anxiety, or other affects. In
general we find that after several memories there is a special and distinct configuration of stimuli regularly present at the moment the tension begins. It is this set of stimuli to which we will later "desensitize"
the person.

When the tension–producing part of the memory is recalled or
relived some people will show signs of anxiety, fear, or anger. As a
general rule, suggestions of relaxation can then be given. For other
subjects—and this is often the case in persons who somatize their conflicts—very little emotion is experienced. In these cases it is often
therapeutically advantageous to give the person verbal feedback to
help increase his emotional awareness. In this way the subject discovers
a new option, that of actually experiencing the emotion which he or
she had previously somatized.

At the end of this memory, which generally takes place over a
period of one to three minutes (although in certain cases it could take
as long as 20 minutes) the subject is told to take a deep breath, let it
out, and as this is done, to let that memory fade away. Further suggestions are given to return the individual to as relaxed a state as that

prior to the memory. It is suggested that memory be erased from his mind for now and not thought about during the remainder of the exploration. Suggestions are then given to take the person back to previous memories which demonstrate the same pattern. Generally the memories in the series are similar to the initial one.

The subject must be observed carefully, especially at the point in the memory at which time the tension begins. Look for signs of anxiety and note what precedes these signs. Such bodily cues as complexion change, lacrimation, turning away of the head, alterations in breathing, gastrointestinal sounds, facial expressions, forehead wrinkling, and other emotive expressions, blushing, and flushing are excellent guides as to the subject's internal state.

Following the second memory, the process is repeated again and again, each time returning to a quiet, relaxed state in which it is suggested that all previous memories be erased for the time being. The number of memories relived and the timespan between memories may vary greatly from individual to individual. As a rough guideline, the third memory may be several years ago, the fourth a decade or two ago, the fifth from the teenage years, the sixth from the preteens, and the seventh back in very early life. Some people never remember anything further back than five or six years. Others may immediately recall a scene from childhood. It is quite possible to obtain an excellent therapeutic response in either case and, in general, there should be no attempt to force a person to go to a stage of his or her life not revealed naturally following permissive suggestion.

Sometimes a subject jumps directly to experiences in early childhood. In such cases it is often helpful to suggest following the early childhood memory: "Now we have seen a way that that pattern took place when you were very young. We will go back to the very early stages of life again in a little while, but now let's go back to some time in the recent past when you had that particular feeling, habit, or symptom." The sequential nature of memories obtained in this way forms a direct link between the behavior pattern occuring now and that occuring back in early childhood.

It is important to separate each of the experiences by suggesting the erasure of prior memories. If this is not done, subjects tend to compare, judge, and analyze instead of experience the memories. If, during a memory, a subject comments, "I feel the same here as I did in the other memory," suggest that he or she erase the other memory and stay in this one.

The scenes to which the subject goes "spontaneously" tend to contain many similar items and patterns—in both stimuli and responses. The same emotion is often experienced in each memory. The subject's way of attempting to solve the problem (e.g. eating candy, withdrawing, etc.) also tends to be repeated.

As each memory is relived, the subject is encouraged to experience fully all aspects of it, including unpleasant emotions and physical symptoms such as nausea. Suggestions are then usually given to "complete the memory" and "erase it."

Since each memory begins with relaxation, goes to a point of maximum emotional intensity, and ends with relaxation again, we are, in a sense, carrying out a desensitization procedure. The subject is finding out—often for the very first time—that this particular emotion or physical reaction can be brought on or released entirely through selective thinking, under his or her own control. Moreover, subjects gain trust in the therapist as they discover that they will not be left to experience pain for hours or days. Instead it becomes clear that after 15 to 30 seconds of experiencing the unpleasant emotion, a suggestion will come which enables them to relax it away. This increase in trust usually leads to deepening of the hypnotic state and further relaxation of resistance and defenses.

As the subject goes through the memories, there are often unclear aspects about which the therapist should ask questions: "What are you feeling?"; "At whom are you angry?"; "How does your stomach feel at this point in the memory?"; "Is anyone else in the room with you?"; "How old are you?" Questions such as these help to clarify stimuli, emotions, and patterns. The fact that the subject is in a relaxed or hypnotized state does not ensure spontaneous selection of all the important facts. Often questions such as these open up whole areas that the subject has been hiding from him– or herself.

EXAMPLES OF SENSITIZING EVENTS

In most cases the "sensitizing event" is no more than a useful fiction. It comes closest to the truth in the exploration of fear reactions which occur in specific settings related to specific stimuli. For example, a woman who had a fear of cats reflected back to many memories in which she had seen cats walking in the street, in friends' houses, or in movies, and was suddenly seized with feelings of panic. In a deeply relaxed state many of these feelings were reproduced in response to her mental imagery, but suggestions of relaxation allowed her to complete the memories, "erase" them, and return to complete relaxation. Finally it was suggested to her: "Go to the very first time in your life that you ever experienced this fear of cats." She then described a very clear memory in which she was standing in the kitchen with her mother, pulling on her mother's apron. She wanted her mother's attention, but her mother was busy talking to a friend. She overheard the friend tell her mother that a neighbor baby had been smothered by a cat that had crawled into its crib. On hearing this, the mother began to cry. The little girl was very confused and very frightened, as she had never seen her mother cry. She was only two years old, but she knew a cat was, and although she wasn't certain what had happened to the baby, she knew that the cat must have done something very terrible to make her mother cry. She relived the feelings (abreacted) as she experienced this memory, In such cases it certainly appears as if there was one event which was "most responsible" for the genesis of a pattern, although in other cases there seems to be a series of events which establishes the pattern.

Although it is very dramatic to have an individual go back through early periods of his life and abreact previously repressed memories, this is neither a necessary nor a sufficient condition for an exploration to be effective. An alcoholic discovered that during each memory his drinking was begun on the night before certain situations in which he feared he might be judged by others, such as going to apply for a job or meeting new people at a dinner party. Once he began drinking he could not stop; months would pass before he again returned to full sobriety. As it turned out, his "sensitizing event" occurred not in childhood, but when he was in the army and had applied for electronics school. The day before the qualifying exam he was very nervous and feared he would fail while his friends would pass. Seeing his discomfort, a well–meaning buddy suggested that he have a few drinks. The tension relief afforded by the drinks was so great that it began a pattern which evolved into a serious drinking problem.

In general, the earlier the memory regressed by the subject, the greater the degree of abreaction, and the greater the degree to which suppressed memories come to the surface, the more fundamental a personality change is possible.

REPRESSED ASPECTS OF MEMORIES

Although in the examples above an entire memory has been re-pressed, more often one finds only certain elements of the memory repressed. A subject who had long considered his mother cruel towards his father came in complaining that he was unfairly treated by his wife, daughters, and other females. In one of his sensitizing events, we discovered an episode in which the father was quite cruel to his mother, followed by her retaliation. Prior to the exploration, the subject has always remembered only a portion of this memory. In this portion he recalled seeing his mother pointing her finger at the door and saying "Get out! Neither I nor the children want you here!" During the exploration, however, the suppressed fragment of the memory reemerged, and with it came the cathartic release of those emotions which the individual had suppressed along with this memory fragment. Following his release, there seemed to be a change in his basic rule of life that "all women are unnecessarily cruel and attack without provocation."

Another subject, an overeater, discovered while reliving recent memories that each episode of overeating was preceded by feelings of deprivation, frustration and an overwhelming desire to consume food, especially ice cream. It was also clear to the therapist that in each one of the situations there was a good deal of withheld anger. In the sensitizing event the subject was five years old, in a hospital crib immediately after a tonsillectomy. She was being offered the ice cream that she had been promised for being "a good girl." Because of the severe pain in her throat, however, she was unable to eat any of it. There were feelings of anger and an inner sense of having been tricked, but because she had no voice she could not express her emotions.

This same constellation of stimuli—feelings of anger and being wronged, feeling of frustration, inability to express feelings, and a yearning for food—had occurred in each of her memories. Prior to this exploration she had often recalled being in the hospital, but all she had ever remembered was standing up in the crib and being unable to eat the ice cream. At no time before had she ever recalled the feeling of being tricked, nor had she ever linked this event to her overeating pattern—even though it was family knowledge that her weight problem began soon after her tonsillectomy. Until this exploration she had been unaware of the feeling of anger that preceded her binges.

Any conceivable element of a sensitizing event can be repressed, including the emotion, one or more of the persons present, the location, inanimate elements in the environment, or physical sensations. Sometimes, however, no repressed memories or memory fragments emerge. In such cases the primary insight is based upon the person's discovery that a particular feeling state regularly precedes a symptom and that there are easily identifiable "stimuli" which can trigger this feeling state.

REWRITING THE SCRIPT

In the ideal case, a clear set of memories leading back to a well–defined sensitizing event appears long before the end of the therapeutic hour and before the second phase, insight and desensitization, begins. About 10 to 20 minutes before the end of the session, the search for new memories is brought to a close with the suggestion, "And on the next visit we will follow this pattern back to an earlier stage in which you will obtain even more insight and relief." Suggestions are then given that the subject to "return to the present," and another moment is spent giving the subject relaxing suggestions to rid the body and mind of any tension which may have developed. Further suggestions are given that the subject not review these memories while relaxing.

The subject is next invited to look at the memory "from your adult perspective." The therapist then assumes the following attitude: "Now you are an adult. As you look back at these memories it will be very obvious to you what mistake in each of the memories that we have been through today but this is understandable now, as you see this whole story laid out in front of you. It is perfectly obvious that this is a pattern that you would never carry out again although you can understand why it had to happen the way it did at those times in the past. You can look at these memories while very relaxed now, even those memories that were frightening a few moments ago." The therapist then reintroduces the subject to the memories, in chronological order, helping through suggestion to maintain relaxation and understanding.

When there has been a particularly large degree of emotional abreaction to certain memories, the subject should be reintroduced to these very gradually. One way of doing this is to suggest that the memories be looked at now as though they were being shown on a television screen located at a distance of 20 feet away. Gradually, as possible, the person imagines the scene replayed at closer and closer range. Ultimately, the individual who experienced a great deal of fear in the original event has the experience of reliving these memories in a relaxed state.

ENCOURAGING INSIGHT

To develop insight into a maladaptive pattern a subject is asked to look at those memories as if they were stories of someone else's life and all that is known about the person. Told to ignore any other memories or characteristic ways of responding to these situations, the subject decides what general suggestions would be given to this person. Other questions help the subject develop insight: "What do you understand now that you didn't understand back in those memories?"; "How would you handle these memories if you were there now?"; "What is the basic pattern that you see as you look at these memories?"; "What do you understand about your symptom now as you look at these memories?"

Insight, when it occurs, is extremely valuable, creating confidence in the technique, trust in the therapist, a positive feeling in the individual, and an intellectual explanation for each to mull over after the session. Occasionally, although an adequate series of memories has evolved, a subject may fail to gain any insight. He or she may not be able to come up with a more adaptive solution or response. In such cases, this suggestion can be given:

> In a moment your subconscious mind is going to give you a word, sentence, or image which is the solution to the problem common to all those memories. It will come to you in the form of a suggestion, and you will find that when you give yourself this suggestion in each of these memories you will be able to handle them much better. At the count of three, you will become aware of that suggestion from your subconscious mind, and you will tell it to me.

At this point the suggestion that occurs may be a rational one such as "Tell my father and mother that I must be independent and have my own thoughts" or "Stand on my own two feet and speed up," or it may be much more abstract such as "Be aware" or even "Call to mind the color green." In one case a subject who had been a heavy smoker was given the suggestion: "In a moment your subconscious mind is going to give you a word or image. Whenever you think about this image you will know that you don't want to smoke anymore." The word "goo" came to him. Later, in his desensitization and future projection experiences, he associated this word with the imaginary experience of finding cigarettes distasteful. It worked well: A two–pack–per–day habit of 30 years' duration ended within six hours with virtually no further desire for a cigarette. Suggestions from the subconscious mind are often the most powerful suggestions that can be given to help change a pattern, probably because they have such great symbolic value for the individual.

With some individuals it may be necessary for the therapist to offer behavioral options:

> I am going to suggest some optional ways of handling these sit-
> uations which you may try if you wish. Imagine yourself, in each
> of these scenes, saying "I'm sorry that you don't like the way I'm
> doing my job, but this is the way I choose to do it." Then feel
> yourself simply relaxing and continuing to do what you know to
> be right, noticing how good it feels to not have tension in your
> body.

Options may be offered more indirectly:

> Is there something you want to tell your mother now that Tommy
> has been given the apple that you earned by scrubbing the floor?
> What do you want to tell your mother as you see her giving Tommy
> the apple that you earned?

The next phase involves suggesting that the subject relive this series of memories again, starting either with the earliest memory and working towards the present, or with the least traumatic memory (especially in the case of phobias):

> Imagine now that you are back in the first memory. This time,
> however, you are going to rewrite the script. As I count from one
> to five, feel yourself going through it in a completely new way—
> a way that leaves you feeling relaxed, confident, in touch with
> your body, centered, secure, and able to express yourself.

The person with a high level of anxiety or fear would simply imagine himself back in these situations without the fear. Those with a habit disorder would imagine themselves walking past the refrigerator, refusing a drink, feeling sick when puffing a cigarette. The individual who had an explosive temper would imagine himself working things out quietly.

In the case of persons with psychosomatic problems diseases with both physical and psychological representations, the presenting symptom acts up at a particular point during each memory and then quiets down again as suggestions of relaxation are given. This is especially true in muscle–tension–related symptoms such as are found in gastrointestinal disorders. An effective deconditioning and mind–body retraining experience occurs when these subjects relive these memories with their bodies feeling totally relaxed. Here, the implicit (or explicit) suggestion is,

> A few moments ago we went through this memory and the body thought that it had to react. As you go through it in a relaxed fashion now your body finds out it does not have to react the way it used to. In the future your subconscious mind will remember this and, in similar situations, instead of reacting as it did the first time through it will respond this new, relaxed way.

THE USE OF CASSETTE TAPES

As the subject is led to relive and rewrite his or her memories, a tape recording is made, recording only certain aspects of the procedure. At the start of the session the relaxation induction is played, but during the actual regression the tape is turned off. As the subject relives each specific memory, general suggestions are given on the tape so that when the subject listens to it at home these suggestions encourage the reliving of other memories which fit the same basic pattern. The theory behind this is that the five or ten memories uncovered in this exploration are merely representatives of perhaps another 20, 100, or 1000 other situations in which the same behavior was carried out. Moreover, even during the days following the exploration, the person will often find the old pattern still cropping up here and there. As the tape is listened to, then the subject has an opportunity to decondition and rewrite these experiences. As specific memories are rewritten by reliving them in mental imagery and changing certain factors in the scene, the subconscious seems to learn the new, more adaptive pattern.

The suggestions on the tape carefully lead the subject through two or three memories of the past, rewriting them. Suggestions are then given to return to the present once again and to begin to look toward the future:

> And now as you look toward the future you find that this new pattern that you have learned will be just as easy to apply as it was a moment ago looking back at the events in the past. Drift forward to some time in the future in which you might ordinarily carry out that unwanted pattern. But as you go through it this time, feel yourself doing it the new way, giving yourself those same suggestions that you did a few moments ago. [The specific suggestions can be mentioned at this point.] As I count from one

to five feel yourself going through this scene handling it just the way you really want to.

The subject is thus led through several such idealized future projections each time he or she listens to the tape. The ultimate effect is that the subject receives a very permissive posthypnotic suggestion that is reinforced each time through the tape. In effect we are suggesting:

> When a similar situation comes up in the future you will always be able to respond as you used to in the past, but this time you will realize that there is a different option that you can choose if you wish. As you go through this scene in the future, feel your ability to be able to choose to eat or not to eat and make the choice that feels right to you now.

Finally, the subject is invited to form an image of the self in a desirable place, doing something that he or she would like to be doing, giving him—or herself the body he or she would like to develop, dressed the way he or she would like to be dressed, moving in a desired and confortable way, using all five senses, and, in effect, creating a perfect self–image. The subject is instructed to feel these strongly, to make the scene real. Suggestions are then given that each time the tape is listened to an old habit pattern will change into a new one, and he or she will become more like an ideal self–image. While this image is being experienced, the suggestion is given that a pleasant feeling within will begin to grow as the therapist counts from one to five, and the subject starts waking up, feeling alert, relaxed, and comfortable. As the subject opens his or her eyes at the count of five, the suggestion is made to take a minute or so just to see how he or she feels.

Often, to avoid the intrusiveness of recording during the session, I will give the patient a copy of a cassette which I have previously prepared. A number of these tapes which contain the entire rescripting process are kept on hand in my office for this purpose.

After the subject's experiences, suggestions are given that the tape be listened to at home, at an average range of two or three times a day for one to three weeks. Persons with high levels of fear usually need more work with the tape. Obviously, if the subject is certain the pattern is completely gone, there is no further need to listen to the tape, although many people will continue to listen just because of the relaxing qualities. Occasionally a patient will feel a continuing sense of discomfort or anxiety even after several listenings. In such cases, its use should be discontinued until further office sessions have explored this problem.

SELECTION OF PATIENTS

Nearly every patient or client receives some benefit from the experience of an exploration. In many cases, even when the presence of irreversible physical changes make it impossible to affect the symptom, the individual has an opportunity to look at it from a relaxed state for the very first time, thus contributing to a perspective that allows him or her to accept and stop struggling against something which cannot be altered. An excellent example of this is provided by the case of a 22–year–old male with a chief complaint of having hands which were "too small." In spite of my informing him that the epiphyses were closed and the bones could not grow, he wished to experience an exploration "just to try." Within a few memories it was clear that his embarrassment was the feeling associated with appearing in public with such small hands, though actually, his hands were normal for his size. The remainder of the memories dealt with earlier childhood experiences of feeling embarrassed and ashamed of himself around others. He was able to "rewrite" these earlier experiences realizing that he was under no real threat and therefore feeling confident. Following this, his anxiety about the size of his hands gradually disappeared. Finally, on his third visit to see me, he told me that he had begun to date girls for the first time and felt quite comfortable about it. He wished no further appointment for therapy as he was not longer concerned about his hands.

In general, individuals who experience an exploration are pleased with an introduction to the relaxed state and find the tape recordings very valuable afterward. There is usually a markedly increased rapport with the therapist regardless of what course subsequent therapy takes.

Several important factors can be outlined which predict how well a particular patient will do. The presenting or "chief" complaint is usually one or more of the following: (1a) maladaptive behavior or habit patterns, (1b) emotional reactions, or (1c) physical symptoms.

Since the exploration deals only with the psychosomatic and not the "organic" aspects of disease processes, good to excellent results have been obtained in working with patients with colitis, gastritis, bruxism, peptic ulcer, chronic indigestion and "gas," headaches—including muscle–contraction (tension) and migraine types, asthma, hyperventilation, hayfever and rhinitis, psychogenic muscle spasm, impotence, and premature ejaculation, female sexual nonresponsiveness, chronic or recurring infections of throat, vagina, and bladder. It has also proven very effective in a number of patients with hypertension, angina pectoris, arthritis (with both diminution of symptoms and return of function), chronic pain (pain usually diminished after the patient's concern about it diminished), cancer, and other "terminal" diseases (individuals were much more able to accept physical limitation and the imminence of death while increasing the quality of their lives), and allergies—especially food and respiratory allergies.

Extremely rapid resolution of symptoms is most common with individuals with phobias and situational fears of less intensity, such as fear of flying, fear of cats, of interviews, of surgery, dentists, schools, tests, etc. Stage fright, fear of interviews, and embarrassment at social functions are also often rapidly resolved.

Another area in which the exploration is most helpful is that of habit disorders. The approach has proven very effective in treating problems of obesity and overeating, habitual episodic alcoholism, smoking, insomnia, drug dependency (including diminishing use of prescription medications), fingernail biting, and other behavioral problems in which the person acts out a pattern that is definitely maladaptive but feels powerless to do anything about it.

This technique, as it focuses on the individual's image–making process, is very useful for self–image problems such as lack of self–confidence, inability to accept a realistic disability (e.g., amputation), excessive guilt, and failure at communication in social and personal situations. Though a longer period of treatment is usually required, it is also useful in the treatment of obsessive worrying, hopelessness, helplessness, mild forms of depression, and incompetence at work.

The exploration is also very effective in mild to moderate psychoneurotic problems (especially those which are associated with an increase in tension or anxiety), loss of temper, periodic depression, chronic maladaptive reactions to family or social–group members, and other reactions which the person links to specific situations.

Results are usually much better when the presenting complaint is experienced in association with a feeling of tension or anxiety.

RESISTANCE TO THERAPY

In general, the longer the problem has been present the more resistant it will be to elimination and more visits will be required. The same holds true when previous treatments have proven unsuccessful, especially when the treatment involved the use of biofeedback, meditation, hypnosis, or psychotherapy, since the somewhat similar features of this prior experience tend to create the expectation of failure. Sometimes, as in the case of overweight, persons who have had many previous dieting failures, may benefit from exploring the feeling of "always being a failure" even before tackling the main symptom of overeating.

The exploration works most rapidly and simply when the presenting symptom is somewhat isolated and is not part of a major personality defense mechanism. For example, a man who underwent an exploration to eliminate a cigar–smoking habit which had resulted in leukoplakia experienced very little change in his pattern. It was noted from his memories that his smoking often occurred in his home and that his wife stayed out of the room whenever he smoked. Soon it became clear in therapy that he had a basic inability to communicate with his wife, and the secondary benefit of keeping her at a distance interfered with the resolution of primary symptom. Following an exploration of his fear of direct communication with people, the habit could be easily eliminated.

SECONDARY GAIN

We must be very aware of the possibility of there being a positive effect or "secondary gain" from symptoms. Very little or no pressure should be exerted when an individual seems to be resistant at any point during the exploration. Often "trading down" may be used. "Is it okay for your headaches to become 50 percent of what they were? 25 percent? 10 percent?" When this and similar maneuvers prove ineffective it is often wise to back off from working on the symptom and to explore the secondary gain. More extensive psychotherapy may sometimes be indicated.

Most individuals in our culture are accustomed to being treated with surgery and drugs—modalities which require little or no cooperation aside from following a simple mechanical instruction. This, of course, is not the case for hypnosis and psychotherapy, for the best technician will fail at such a technique as the selective awareness exploration if the subject refuses to cooperate. Cooperation, in this case, means that the client or patient allows himself to follow instructions in a relaxed way and to report on images and memories that occur. It is also helpful if the individual is willing to accept some responsibility for changing his or her own patterns. Yet, there are those who find even this modicum of cooperation to be difficult. If at any point resistance is noticed, it is best dealt with immediately, before the therapist finds himself maneuvered into a "no–win" situation.

CONCLUSION

The selective awareness exploration, then, is an approach through which a presenting symptom can serve as a convenient starting point for therapy. This approach involves the teaching of relaxation and desensitization techniques, the development of a cognitive framework within which the patient can be helped to view the symptom as a part of a style of response, and the encouragement of individual acceptance of responsibility for selecting a new, more adaptive response pattern. The use of desensitization and rescripting techniques can be self–applied, using meditative/autogenic/self–hypnotic modalities. Clinical experience suggests that the approach is effective in a broad range of problems.

REFERENCES

1. Cheek, D., & LeCron, L. *Clinical hypnotherapy.* New York: Grune & Stratton, 1968.
2. Korger, W. *Clinical and experimental hypnosis.* Philadelphia: Lippincott, 1963.
3. Meares, W., & Ainslie, W. *A system of medical hypnosis.* New York: Saunders, 1960.
4. Wolpe, J. *Psychotherapy by reciprocal inhibition.* Stanford, California: Stanford University Press, 1958.
5. Miller, E. *Rehearsal for reality—relaxation, imagery and healing.* Audio Cassette available from The Source, Menlo Park, California. Miller
6. Miller, E. *Feeling Good.* Englewood Cliffs, New Jersey: Prentice–Hall. 1978.
7. Miller, E. *Writing your own script.* Self–teaching audiocassette tape. Available from E. Miller, P.O. Box W, Stanford, Ca. 94305.
8. Miller, E. *Applications of autosuggestion.* An experiential introduction. Cassette tape available from E. Miller, P.O. Box W, Stanford, Ca. 94305.
9. Erickson, M., Rossi E., and Rossi S., *Hypnotic realities.* Text and audio cassette. New York: Irvington, 1976.

Chapter 4

GUIDED IMAGERY:

Healing Through the Mind's Eye

Dennis T. Jaffe, Ph.D.
David E. Bresler, Ph.D.

The use of personal mental images to diagnose and modify bodily processes is an ancient part of the healing tradition. The healer/physician/shaman/priest has always utilized the latent power of the imagination to alter the body, and many traditional health–care systems have focused on the amazing power of the mind to promote the healing process.[1-3] Recent demonstrations that the autonomic nervous system can be modified through learning and various cognitive strategies have encouraged contemporary health practitioners to begin exploring the applications of therapeutic guided imagery.

COMMUNICATING WITH THE BODY

Guided imagery is a method of communicating with autonomic physiological processes which occur outside of conscious awareness. This internal exchange of information can proceed in two directions. First, information about subtle physiological processes can be brought to conscious awareness as an aid to diagnosis. Secondly, the power of the imagination can be recruited to promote specific physiological changes as an aid to therapy. Within limits yet to be determined, the conscious mind, utilizing mental imagery, participates in both types of communication.

We have suggested elsewhere that there are two fundamentally different higher order languages utilized by the nervous system for internal communication.[4] Verbal thoughts most directly access the somatic nervous system, so if, for example, you wish to stand up, all you need to do is think "stand up now" and your voluntary nervous system will coordinate the appropriate muscular activity. On the other hand, the language of imagery directly accesses the *autonomic nervous system* (ANS), which regulates breathing, the heartbeat, blood chemistry, digestion, tissue regeneration and repair, immune and inflammatory responses, and many other bodily functions essential to life.

To illustrate the differing effects of verbal command and imagery over "involuntary" functions, we often use the following demonstration:

> First, using verbal language, order yourself to "manufacture and secrete saliva." By thinking about this command, see how much saliva you can generate. Most people produce a little, but not much, for the parts of the body that produce saliva do not respond well to verbal commands.
>
> Mental imagery represents a different approach to physiological change. Imagine that you have in your hand a big, yellow, juicy lemon. Visualize it in your mind's eye until you smell its fresh tartness. Then imagine taking a knife, and slicing into the lemon. Carefully cut out a thick, juicy section. Now, take a deep bite of your imaginary lemon and begin to sense that tart, sour lemon juice splashing in your mouth, saturating every taste bud of your tongue so fully that your lips and cheeks curl. Swirl it in your mouth for an other 15 to 20 seconds, bathing every corner of your mouth with its acid taste.

If you were able to paint the suggested picture vividly in your mind's eye, the image probably produced substantial salivation, for the autonomic nervous system easily understands and responds to the language of imagery. It is a short step to hypothesize that other physiological functions—including those directly concerned with the body's resistance to disease—may also be mobilized via imagery.

The need for a therapeutic approach to the use of mental imagery is suggested by the fact that patients are always using imagery to send messages to the body—messages which in many cases may inhibit the healing process. For example, many patients with chronic pain picture themselves as helpless, hopeless victims of an incurable illness. In their mind's eye, they focus on such thoughts as, "I hurt so much . . . I am so limited by this pain (or disease) . . . I feel terrible . . . No doctor can help me . . . This can only get worse . . ." When the imagination is preoccupied by these negative pictures, the autonomic nervous system is being told, in effect, "Prepare the body to be helpless. Don't even bother mobilizing the immune and inflammatory defenses that might facilitate healing. Just give up." It's not surprising, then, that these patients often don't get better, as these messages become a self–fulfilling prophecy.

Images seem to have a very literal effect on the body. No matter what types of medical terminology are used to describe a specific diagnosis, if a patient experiences discomfort as "a sizzling hot poker constantly being stabbed into my neck," as "a lion gnawing on my back, tearing deeper into the nerves with very bite," or as "wringing out the nerves like they're a wet washcloth," then these are the ways it will be most fully experienced.

A single mental picture, then, can be far more potent than a dictionary of words. Thus many clinicians have begun to use positive images to help their patients heal themselves. For example, while sitting in a dentist's chair, a patient can be taught to stop his or her gums from bleeding by creating a vivid image of it actually happening. Several dentists have reported that when they ask their patients to imagine that freezing–cold ice was being applied to their bleeding gums, the patients reported that the area soon became numb. In addition, the blood vessels constricted, and the bleeding stopped. In a similar way, the effectiveness of medication can often be enhanced through imagery. For example, a patient taking antibiotics for an ear infection can be taught to imagine that the blood vessels nourishing the ear are becoming dilated. This may permit more blood—and a greater concentration of the antibiotic—to flow into the ear, hastening the healing process.

All physical symptoms and illnesses are to some degree affected by the mind. Healing can thus be enhanced by positive and helpful images and expectations, and hampered and slowed by depression, hopelessness, and fatigue. In our opinion, the way a person uses his or her mind is a critical factor in the outcome of therapy.

This is true whatever the cause of illness. For example, even if a person is recovering from an operation after an accident, or has an illness caused by some hereditary predisposition (with little stress–related or behavior–related etiology), the recovery process can still be speeded up or slowed down by the use of mental imagery. In this way guided imagery represents an important adjunctive technique for nearly all other forms of medical treatment.

DIAGNOSTIC USE OF IMAGERY

One of the most difficult aspects of medical diagnosis is an accurate assessment of the patient's internal perceptions and expectations. Imagery can be most helpful in this regard, for it is a highly evocative language that comprehensively conveys unconscious attitudes and processes. As part of the diagnostic interview, a patient can be asked to close his or her eyes and to allow the mind to present a picture that represents the experience of the problem. The patient is then instructed to draw the picture that came to mind as accurately as possible.

These pictures can lead to important information not only about the illness, but also about the patient's beliefs, hopes, expectations, and fears about the body, its ability to withstand the illness, and the effectiveness of the recommended treatment. Many patients have uncannily accurate intuitions about their illnesses, and the imagery process can make these available to the diagnostician adding to other sources of information.

One of our hypertensive patients pictured himself crushed by a huge vise. A woman drew her chronic bronchitis as a plug in her chest blocking her breath. A man envisioned his added weight as in inner tube keeping him afloat on a stormy sea. A woman's lymph cancer was pictured as a termite invasion. Such pictures offer a first glimpse of the psychic reality which is associated with a symptom. In symbolizing this reality through pictures, patients often open psychological doors that permit them and their therapists to explore the meaning of their symptoms in ways previously unavailable.

Patients can also be asked to create a new and different image, adding or to altering the original picture with something that inspires and promotes the healing process. For example, a man with an ulcer who pictured his stomach as being punctured with arrows drew a heart and a pathway from it to his stomach. Discussing the picture, he began to examine his lack of intimate relationships with others, his denial of needs for companionship, and his characterization of himself as a "loner." He was lonely and needed to open his heart to others.

The imagery a patient chooses can be based on his knowledge of the actual physiological processes through which the body combats illness, or on a fanciful or symbolic representation of how it might happen. For example, one cancer patient utilized the following image:

> I'd begin to visualize my cancer as I saw it in my mind's eye. I'd make a game of it. The cancer would be a snake, a wolverine, or some vicious animal. The cure—white, husky dogs by the millions. It would be a confrontation of good and evil. I'd envision the dogs grabbing the cancer and shaking it, ripping it to shreds. The forces of good would win. The cancer would shrink—from a big snake to a little snake—and then disappear. Then the white army of dogs would lick up the residue and clean my abdominal cavity until it was spotless.

Several interesting observations concerning the relationship between imagery and the prognosis of treatment for cancer patients have been described by the Simontons.[5] From the nature of the image a person selects, they have predicted with some accuracy how well that individual will fare in treatment. The Simontons were not the first to note how a person's symbolic reality mirrors the physical disease. Researcher Bruno Klopfer[6] was almost unerringly able to predict from Rorschach responses which patients had slow or fast growing tumors. Images seem to yield important diagnostic indications about a patient's deep unconscious attitudes about the self and the illness.

The Simontons compare the patient's image of his body's power with that of the cancer. Generally, the stronger side in the image prevails. If the cancer is pictured as a dangerous animal, and the white cells as puffs of snow or cotton, the prognosis is poor. As an example, the Simontons note that people who spontaneously choose an image of ants to represent their cancer seem to do poorly. They relate this to the real difficulty in attempting to eradicate every single ant in a plague of ants. In their residential treatment program, the Simontons work with their patients' imagery to alter or modify the images as well as their attitudes so that the cancer does, in fact, lose the mental battle.

The symbols a person chooses to represent physical processes thus often present accurate, important diagnostic information about the actual state of the body. The goal of the diagnostician is to make this inner information clear, explicit and relevant to the treatment process.

THERAPEUTIC USE OF IMAGERY

It is a short step from the diagnostic use of imagery to its therapeutic application. If a patient presents a negative, helpless, or hopeless picture of the illness or the body's potential for overcoming it, helping that individual see the situation more positively may have a significant effect on response to treatment.

The most common therapeutic use of mental imagery is in the induction of what is known as the "relaxation response." Relaxation is a well-known antidote to excessive daily stress and its result is chronic activation of the sympathetic nervous system. The relaxation state—characterized by parasympathetic dominance, muscle relaxation, and slowed respiration—is entered by the induction of mental images that suggest physical regeneration and deep rest. There are as many types of relaxation training as there are over-the-counter medications, ranging from transcendental meditation to progressive relaxation, autogenic training, meditation, and self-hypnosis, but they all seem to utilize the same basic principles to initiate the relaxation response.

A person cannot enter the relaxation state by merely telling his body to relax. Since the relaxation response is triggered by the ANS, this verbal language alone would be ineffective. Indeed, the more one tries to relax, the more the muscles tighten, and the less relaxed one becomes. The relaxation response is attained by creating a mental image of a scene, in which one is deeply relaxed, or by suggesting via imagery certain changes in the body which stimulate the relaxation state. For example, repeating to oneself the phrase "I am at peace," or simply paying attention to one's breathing, letting all other thoughts quietly slip away, are two ways to initiate this state. We often ask patients simply to remember a wonderful vacation spot where they were totally relaxed and at peace. The memory stimulates the body to reexperience the relaxation response.

Attaining a state of bodily relaxation is a prerequisite for all work with therapeutic guided imagery, for it provides inhibition of somatic muscle activity and verbal thoughts and allows mental images to become dominant. The relaxation response can usually be induced using any of the currently popular methods,[7,8] and for the minority of patients who have difficulty in attaining this state, biofeedback training may also be helpful.

Once a state of deep relaxation is entered, the patient is individually guided to create a picture in the mind's eye of what he or she wishes the body to do. For the medically sophisticated or the technically minded, the image can be a precise representation of the desired physiological change. For example, a person might want the liver to produce an extra supply of a particular enzyme or the immune system to increase the number of white cells. Many people like to read medical texts to find out how their body might aid in the healing process.

Even symbolic or fanciful images can be helpful. Several physicans who have used these methods feel that the healing image doesn't have to be realistic for it to be effective. Thus, patients who imagine little men with ray guns charging through the body killing an oozy green virus may achieve the same beneficial results.

An account of how mental imagery can be integrated into a medical treatment program was given to us by a nurse born with a hip deformity who learned to control her continual pain by a variety of methods without restricting her activities. She began by paying attention to the particular needs of various parts of her body, especially her hips and legs. When she felt discomfort, she would ask her tight legs or muscles what she could do to take care of them. "Massage us," or "take a day off and rest," they would reply through what she felt was a voice in her head. If she needed to do something particularly difficult or especially active, such as like a day of sailing, she would strike a bargan: "If you let me do this without much pain, I will in return take special care to rest you for the next two days. Is that all right?", she might ask, and wait for an affirmative reply. By becoming intimately aware of the needs of her hips and joints, and by catering to them, she was able to enjoy 15 active, relatively pain–free, productive years, until the total hip replacement operation was developed and recommended to her.

She then began preparing for a difficult highly experimental procedure which was fraught with potential hazards. Several times a day, she imagined what her body needed to do. She told her blood vessels not to rupture and her immune system how to react. She prepared her body for each step of the procedure over and over in her mind's eye.

She also imaged the operation going perfectly well. She imagined the surgeons being totally relaxed and their hands being swift and sure. She imagined that they had had a relaxing weekend and were refreshed and optimistic about her operation, scheduled for a Monday morning. While her imaginings may not have had much effect on the hospital personnel, it helped to calm her and increase her optimism about the outcome. In effect, she prepared her whole body by way of imagery for the difficult process to come.

Despite all her preparation, however, a small complication developed during the generally successful operation. One of the nerves in her leg was damaged, leaving her with no feeling along part of the leg. She was initially frustrated, but soon got to work. She spent every moment she could imagining the nerve growing and becoming whole. Her physician said that it might grow a millimeter a day and that she had to grow it along her whole leg. She imagined it going ever faster, and, slowly, over months, normal sensations did return. Her story demonstrates how imagery and relaxation can become an integral part of traditional medicine and perhaps increase the chances of success in high–risk medical and surgical procedures.

This account also illustrates another important therapeutic use of imagery, namely, the use of positive future images to activate positive physical changes. Imagining a positive future outcome is an important technique for countering the initial negative images, beliefs, and expectations a patient may have. In essence, it transforms a negative palcebo effect (or nocebo) into a positive one. Positive self–guided imagery also helps by giving the patient something active and constructive to do.

The use of positive images to reinforce health has been an integral part of many healing traditions. Around the turn of the century, Emile Coué, a French pharmacist, opened a clinic in which positive imagery was used as a method of attaining maximum health. His famous phrase, which his patients repeated to themselves several times a day, was the simple, "Every day, in every way, I am becoming better and better." That basic suggestion, combined with specific formulae for specific ailments, was aimed at using imagery and suggestion to affect physiological responses. Coué believed that imagining an outcome would do far more to bring it about than willing, or forcing oneself, to do something. Imagination was a gentle guide, taking the body in the direction of its wanderings.

By imagining the end point one seeks—full health, some specific career or life goal—without willing it or forcing oneself to desire it, the mind is carried in that direction. This is especially important when a person may be imagining or expecting a negative outcome. The power of positive suggestion plants a seed which redirects the mind— through the mind and the body—toward a positive goal. Using phrases and positive thoughts regularly as part of a routine relaxation process is one of the best ways to weaken the power of negative images.

In addition to creating healing images, patients are asked to create a set of positive phrases that they tend to forget or feel they would like to remember and to write them on a card. They then place the card on their bathroom mirror and try to repeat the phrases to themselves from time to time during the day. People create suggestions such as, "I can get the love I want without having to eat," or "I will feel tremendous, vital, healthy, and breathe freely each day that I do not smoke" or "I will treat my body with love and respect."

Such messages help to counteract negative patterns that may have been set inadvertently years before and which subconsciously set in motion negative physiological cycles which can culminate in illness or cause health–destructive behavior. Many people also find it helpful to add affirmative personal statements, letting themselves know that they are worthy of being healthy, of being loved, or of changing in a positive direction to reach some of their life goals.

THE INNER ADVISER: A DIAGNOSTIC AND THERAPEUTIC USE OF IMAGERY

Clinicians are experimenting with many creative and highly experimental uses of mental imagery. One of the most dramatic techniques we have used involves what is known as "the inner adviser." This technique was popularized by Irving Oyle[9] and Mike Samuels[10] and is utilized by many practitioners of Integral Medicine. By creating and interacting with an inner adviser, a person learns to gather important information from the subconscious, and is able to feel comfortable and familiar with parts of themselves previously inaccessible to conscious awareness.

A good illustration of this technique is the case of Julie, whose life changed suddenly one afternoon. Until then, she had been miserable and confused tormented by a grinding, throbbing pain in her lower back that had persisted for nearly six years. At its worst, the discomfort radiated into other parts of her body as well, razor–sharp bullets firing into her shoulders, chest, and buttocks. To aggravate things even further, her marriage had collapsed, and she felt ravaged by the strain of raising her teenage sons by herself.

But one afternoon, during a period of relaxation in a therapeutic session, Julie learned how to contact her inner adviser—an imaginary living creature—in her subconscious mind. During Julie's first experience with this technique, she imagined she was in a beautiful wooded forest and soon made contact with an imaginary hummingbird.

> DOCTOR: What is the hummingbird's name?
> JULIE: Sam.
> DOCTOR: Tell Sam you mean him no harm, that you would just like to meet with him occasionally to talk things over with him. Would that be okay?
> JULIE: He says he'd be willing to do that.
> DOCTOR: Good. Tell him you have brought some honey and water for him today. And ask him if there is any advice he'd like to give you in return.

JULIE: He says yes.
DOCTOR: What does he want to tell you?
JULIE: He says he wants me to start liking myself more and
filling my life with more fun.

Later in the exercise, Julie was told to try the following experiment:

DOCTOR: Ask Sam, as a demonstration of his friendship
and good faith, if he is willing to take away your pain right
now, even for just a moment. . . . Will he do that?
JULIE: Yes, he says he will.

Within seconds, Julie's pain was gone. It stayed away for several hours. The sore and aching muscles that had plagued her for so long were finally free of discomfort. By the time Julie's pain returned, later that day, her disposition had improved remarkably. For the first time in years, she realized that it was possible for her to be pain–free. In the ensuing weeks, she continued to communicate with her adviser, who helped her to start thinking more positively about her own future. After a few weeks, she was progressing very well toward controlling her pain completely.

The advisers that such people as Julie create from the inner recesses of her unconscious mind can also create change in subconscious belief systems. Earlier we noted that patients may become imprisoned by their own inappropriate belief systems. This happens not only on the conscious level but subconsciously as well. Indeed, quite unknowingly, a patient may envision him– or herself as a hopeless, helpless victim of pain. It then becomes essential to become aware of that self-created vision, and to adopt a new belief system that will facilitate healing. The adviser technique can help a person become intimately connected with the subconscious mind and aid in the incorporation of new beliefs, new expectations, and new habits.

In the process, communication with the adviser also fosters a "centering process," in which one's ability to observe the intuitive side becomes very sophisticated. Long after the immediate physical problem has been resolved, sensitivity to the activities of the subsconscious mind can continue if contact with the adviser is maintained.

Not only has guided imagery proven immensely valuable, but most patients are quite receptive to the technique. They—and we—have learned that guided imagery is basically just a way of talking to oneself, of acknowledging and making use of intuition.

People sometimes find themselves reacting to a particular event by saying, "Damn, I knew that was going to happen!" How did they know? Of course, it was the intuitive part of the mind—in essence, an inner adviser—that told them. The adviser is simply the imaginary embodiment in human or animal form, of subconscious intuition and knowledge.

Getting in touch with an adviser is an extension of the imagery techniques we have already described. First, a person enters the relaxation state. Then, he or she imagines being in a place with the perfect calm and comfort of home. In this special healing place will he or she meet an adviser. After spending a few moments enjoying and relaxing in this special place, the person then sits back and waits for the adviser to appear. Instructed to avoid trying consciously to create someone or something, the person lets the spontaneous creativity and wisdom of the subconscious come up with an image which embodies a benevolent guide or adviser.

It is important to wait until the adviser appears in human, animal, or other life form. Since the symbolic range is enormous, each person creates an adviser in a form uniquely suited to his or her inner image of helpfulness. When the adviser arrives, the person is asked to greet it and to begin the process of getting to know the adviser. This might include introducing him– or herself and learning the adviser's name. It might also include an exchange of gifts. Then the process of dialogue and interaction begins. The person talks to the adviser, who answers either directly or sometimes with metaphorical ambiguity or other indirect messages. People usually have the experience of receiving surprising or unexpected information from this inner oracle, and the information received is usually of critical importance to their healing process.

This seemingly silly process of creative imagination is a way to give concrete form and substance to subconscious feelings, attitudes, and stored information. Patients are asked to talk regularly with their advisers, and as they practice this technique they find that they can discover increasingly important sources of inner guidance.

Once a person has an adviser—whether cat, squirrel, deer, or dolphin—he or she can discuss anything on his or her mind, or anything that the adviser might like to talk about. There are no limits, except that the dialogue should be kept totally honest on both sides. The adviser provides an endless number of insights—not only about a person's pain or illness but about other aspects of life as well.

In working with hundreds of patients using this guided imagery technique, we find that the adviser can be helpful in at least four distinct ways.

1. *The adviser can provide advice on how to reduce stress and pain.* When a patient needs pain relief or stress reduction, he can ask his adviser for suggestions. The adviser plays the role of an "imaginary doctor," as Samuels and Bennett note.[10] We often ask patients to talk their physical problems over with this make–believe doctor, or adviser. For example, Sylvia, an ulcer victim with terrible stomach pains, described a meeting with Shorty, her adviser, and the surprising revelation she received: "Shorty's sweet and darling, and the last time I talked with him, he said I needed to keep my pain for a while longer so I'll continue working on myself. He said if I didn't have pain, I'd quit the relaxation exercise and become too anxious again. When I've learned to relax myself more consistently, he says, the pain will go away."

2. *The adviser can provide support and protection.* An adviser can supply encouragement for decisions already made sometimes with greater enthusiasm and support than found among friends or family members. The adviser can also shield a person from danger by warning him in advance when he or she is about to do something that is not in his or her best interest. It is like having a personal oracle.

3. *The adviser has the power to give total and complete symptomatic relief.* One way the adviser can demonstrate power is by providing total symptomatic relief for a few moments. Once the adviser's powers are recognized in essence, as his or her own, then begins an understanding of the patient's enormous control over his or her own body and health.

4. *The adviser can help discover the message behind symptoms.* Because symptoms are a message that something is wrong, it is essential for a patient to identify that message if wishing to completely overcome a problem. Often, a message has been repressed, and is not available to the conscious mind. But the adviser can help to uncover it in a gentle, loving, nonthreatening way. An adviser can tell not only why the body hurts but also why the person's whole life doesn't feel right.

After a patient has developed a strong relationship with an adviser, we recommend that other advisers be sought out as well. We suggest that patients invite their advisers to bring mates or other acquaintances to the next meeting. Some people use several advisers to help resolve a particular conflict they may be experiencing. Two advisers can debate the issue, taking opposing viewpoints, while the individual is able to evaluate their respective positions objectively.

Terry, a UCLA Pain Control Unit patient, was suffering from chronic endometriosis (inflammation of the inner lining of the uterus). She asked her first adviser, a dog named Max, to recruit two other advisers to discuss her indiscriminant sexual activities, which she thought might be contributing to her problem. One of the new advisers was a rabbit named Rachel, who told Terry, "You live only once, and life is very short. Why not make it as sweet as you can? Have as many different sexual experiences as possible and don't worry about attachments. Just live loose and free!"

The other adviser was a deer named Bambi, who argued, "You have to respect yourself before others will respect you. Rather than having a lot of meaningless experiences, save yourself for the right person. It's quality, not quantity that's important."

Terry felt that she received some very helpful insights from this debate. In a subsequent meeting with all three of her advisers, she decided she wanted to be more like the deer than the rabbit and that while she still might occasionally allow herself to be sexually free (as the rabbit), it would never again be a permanent lifestyle.

We feel that the advisers represent dialogues between different parts of one's nervous system. Although a patient may feel, "I'm just talking to myself. How can that help me?", it's the unique content and symbolism of the dialogue that is important. We ask, "Why did only certain responses pop into your head? Why did your adviser assume the name Roger? Why was he a frog? Why did he tell you to love yourself more? All of these have relevance and meaning to your life."

CONCLUSION

The use of inner advisers, healing imagery, positive suggestion, relaxation training, and diagnostic imagery as part of medical practice represents a departure from the orthodox conception of the doctor's role but is very much in keeping with the traditional conception and practice of the healer. Mental imagery mobilizes the latent, inner powers of the person, which have immense potential to aid in the healing process and in the promotion of health. The techniques we have described are easy to teach and easy to learn and have no negative side effects, so that in many ways they make an ideal adjunct to any other type of therapy. It is our hope that health professionals from all disciplines will begin to utilize them to help their patients more effectively help themselves.

REFERENCES

1. Beecher, H.K. The powerful placebo. *Journal of the American Medical Association.* 1955, *151,* 1602–1606.
2. Cousins, N. The mysterious placebo. *Saturday Review,* October 1, 1977, pp. 9–16.

3. Frank, J. The faith that heals. *John Hopkins University Medical Journal,* 1975, *137,* 127–131.
4. Bresler, D.E. & Trubo, R. *Free yourself from pain.* New York: Simon & Schuster, 1979.
5. Simonton, O.C., Matthews–Simonton, S., & Creighton, J. *Getting well again.* Los Angeles, Ca.: Tarcher, 1978.
6. Klopfer, B. Psychological variables in human cancer. *Journal of Projective Techniques,* 1957, *21,* 337–339.
7. White, J., & Fadiman, J. *Relax.* New York: Dell Publishing Company, 1976.
8. Bresler, D. Conditioned relaxation: The pause that refreshes. This volume, Chapter 5.
9. Oyle, I. *Time, space and the mind.* Millbrae, Ca.: Celestial Arts, 1976.
10. Samuels, M., & Bennett, H. *The well body book.* New York: Random House/Bookworks, 1973.

A PREVENTIVE APPROACH TO BEHAVIORAL MEDICINE:

Biofeedback and Beyond

Kenneth R. Pelletier, Ph.D.

Stress is an integral element in the biological scheme of living organisms. All have innate stress alarm reactions which enable them to cope effectively with their environments. Hans Selye[1] has suggested that stress is "the rate of wear and tear within the body" or, more abstractly, "the state manifested by a specific syndrome which consists of all the nonspecifically induced changes within a biologic system." Two of the most fundamental characteristics of life, self–preservation and procreation, could not be realized without the innate stress mechanisms.

For people living in sophisticated, postindustrial western cultures, however, stress often becomes excessive and deleterious. Modern men and women have developed a social and economic structure and a sense of time urgency which subject them to more and greater stress than at any time in human history.[2]

Stress affects both sexes and all ages. People in late adolescence begin to accumulate effects of stress though this may not manifest until their forties or fifties. Some people are vaguely aware that their personal stress is taking a heavy health toll. Others are sure it is and have the medical bills as evidence.

Many of the major environmental triggers of stress are readily apparent. Negative events, such as financial difficulties, a death in the family, a violation of the law, or a foreclosure on a loan are immediately recognizable as severe stressors. However, not all stress arises in negative circumstances. Recent longitudinal studies appear to show that events which most people consider positive or pleasurable can be as stress–inducing as those that are considered negative.[3] Positive occurrences such as marriage, a promotion, a desired pregnancy, an outstanding personal achievement, or even a vacation can be stressors. These events require a person to adapt or change and they tax his or her physical and mental adaptive mechanisms just as negative stressors do. When too many adjustments must be made in a brief period of time, tension and stress are the results.

It is important, however, to differentiate between injurious and noninjurious stress responses. Obviously, not all stress can or should be avoided. A normal adaptive stress reaction occurs when the source of stress is identifiable and clear. When this particular challenge is met, an individual returns to a level of normal functioning relatively quickly. However, when several sources exist simultaneously, the individual cannot return to a normal psychological or physiological baseline as rapidly, and the stress reaction persists. This persisting stress reaction may be implicated in many psychosomatic disorders.

The precise processes by which excessive stress induces illness are clearly defined in some stress–related diseases and poorly understood in others. Consciously or unconsciously, perceived stressors alter neurophysiological activity, endocrine and immunological balance, blood supply and pressure, respiratory rate and pattern, and digestive processes. Whether the physiological changes resulting from stress are recognized or not, they may significantly affect a person's resistance to disease and create damage in their own right.

Standard medical texts attribute anywhere from 50 to 80 percent of all disease to psychosomatic or stress–related origins.[4] Even the most conservative sources classify the following illnesses as pyschosomatic: peptic ulcer, mucous colitis, ulcerative colitis, bronchial asthma, atopic dermatitis, urticaria and angioneurotic edema, hay fever, arthritis, Raynaud's disease, hypertension, hyperthyroidism, amenorrhea, enuresis, paroxysmal tachycardia, migraine headache, impotence, a variety of sexual dysfunctions, sleep–onset insomnia, alcoholism, and a range of neurotic and psychotic disorders. Hypertension alone affects 20 to 25 million people in the United States and predisposes its victims to such lethal consequences as arteriosclerosis, congestive heart failure, and stroke.

There is also a tendency for individuals to regard normal stress reactions as abnormal, and thereby aggravate the stress. Such reactions may also be strongly implicated in the genesis of psychosomatic disorders. Neurologist A. T. W. Simeons in an excellent book, *Man's Presumptuous Brain*, analyzes this process or "psychosomatic onset."

> When these once normal and vitally important reactions to fear do reach his conscious awareness, he interprets them as something abnormal and regards them as afflictions . . . These now largely useless reactions, and their misinterpretation as signs of disease, produce a new, this time conscious, state of alarm: the dread of disease . . . It is in this way that the vicious cycles which cause psychosomatic disease become established.[5]

The genesis of a psychosomatic disorder can be described as follows. An individual is confronted with a stressful situation which seems impossible to resolve. The individual then makes an unconscious choice which allows him or her to cope with the irresolvable situation. He or she develops a psychosomatic disorder, such as a migraine headache, so severely and incapacitating that the person is released from the responsibilities weighing so heavily. Symptoms allow a person to remove him– or herself from an untenable situation from which he or she cannot extricate by any other means. Anthropologist Gregory Bateson[6] has termed this kind of predicament in which an individual must choose between two equally unacceptable alternatives a "double–bind situation."

The sympton frees the individual from the necessity of dealing with the complex and unmanageable stress situation. Once ill, peers and family modify their expectations and demands. Illness postpones, or perhaps even prevents, a confrontation with the problematic situation. Once this course of action is taken and proves successful, there is a tendency on the part of the person to reinitiate the same pattern of behavior in response to future stressors. Unfortunately, the decision which leads to the development of disease in response to stress is usually made at an unconscious level, and the symptomatic response patterns may continue far beyond the point at which they are an effective means of dealing with stress.

There is an extensive body of research which strongly suggests that specific personality types are predisposed to develop particular kinds of psychosomatic disorder. Among the most comprehensive research is that of Meyer Friedman and Ray Rosenman, cardiologists at Mt. Zion Hospital in San Francisco. After years of working with cardiovascular patients, they were able to delineate a well–defined behavior pattern in their patients. Typical heart patients were noted to be impatient, aggressive, extremely goal–oriented, ambitious, restless, and always under time pressure even when supposedly "relaxing." Friedman and Rosenman termed this pattern "Type A" behavior and reported their research in *Type A Behavior and Your Heart*.[7] Research by others suggests that other personality types may be particularly vulnerable to such conditions as cancer and migraine headaches.[8,9]

Present therapeutic interventions for psychosomatic disorders are far from encouraging. Treatment of hypertension, for example, usually involves the prescription of one or more drugs to regulate blood pressure. The cost, disturbing side effects, and necessity of long, continued dependence on medication make chemotherapy less than satisfactory. Similarly, the stress which predisposes one to the variety of psychosomatic illnesses is also dealt with chemically. Each year approximately 144 million prescriptions are written for psychotropic drugs including antidepressants and minor and major tranquilizers, which may have disconcerting and dangerous side effects. If we continue to prescribe at the same increasing rate, psychiatrist Barry Blackwell[10] expects "that with the arrival of the millenium, in 2000, the whole of America will be taking tranquilizers."

As time goes on, and as the number of Americans suffering from stress–related disorders increases, it becomes increasingly important to find nonpharmacological means to treat and prevent these conditions.

CLINICAL BIOFEEDBACK

At present a number of new therapies are being used to treat and prevent stress disorders. Some techniques, such as meditation, are ancient; others, such as biofeedback, are new. All—including autogenic training, progressive relaxation, various types of classical meditation, yoga, and clinical biofeedback—are helping people to adjust to stress. They operate in two major ways: (1) through instructing individuals in achieving deep relaxation, a state which serves as a prophylaxis against the development of stress–related disorders, and (2) by teaching people to exercise a control over their autonomic or involuntary physiological functions, which only ten years ago was considered impossible. So far, biofeedback is the most widely used and carefully resarched of these techniques.

Biofeedback is based upon three basic principles: (1) that any neurophysiological or other biological function which can be monitored and amplified by electronic instrumentation and instantaneously fed back to a person through any one of his five senses can be regulated by that individual; (2) "every change in the physiological state is accompanied by an appropriate change in the mental emotional state, conscious or unconscious, and conversely, every change in the mental emotional state, conscious or unconscious, is accompanied by an appropriate change in the physiological state[11] and (3) a meditative state of deep relaxation is conducive to the establishment of voluntary control by allowing the individual to become aware of internal imagery, fantasies, and sensations.

Research and clinical practice with biofeedback and meditation have demonstrated that many autonomic or involuntary nervous–system functions can be brought under conscious control if an individual has information about the process. Actually, there is no such thing as controlling a biological function; training only helps elicit certain subjective states to be detected and manipulated through subjective feelings, focus of attention, and thought processes. The functions that may be obtained when these subjective states are elicited include brainwaves, heart rate and regularity, muscle tension, blood flow, and (in experimental work) stomach acidity and single nerve impulses.

At the present time, a great deal of the clinical work in biofeedback is oriented toward the alleviation of pathology. However, treating specific symptoms with certain feedback modalities is but a limited application of biofeedback. In a larger context, its greatest value may lie in its ability to introduce people to a relaxation response which can help them to reduce daily stress prior to the development or diagnosis of a psychosomatic disorder. To accomplish this, biofeedback technology is combined with meditation, other relaxation techniques and a variety of psychotherapeutic procedures. Such combinations enable clinicians to help their patients to rely on their own awareness and understanding of internal states as they develop, rather than on the electronic instruments, appropriate only after revealed symptoms become fixed.

Though clinical biofeedback can be used in well–developed illnesses, most positive results are usually obtained with people seeking clinical help for minor symptoms. These people learn to alleviate their symptoms, and overcome habitual chronic stress responses, thereby prevent the occurrence of more severe disorders. In referring to stress–related disorders, George B. Whatmore and Daniel R. Kohli[12] have used the term "dysponesis" (from "dys" meaning wrong or faulty and "ponos" meaning effort or energy). Biofeedback instrumentation is designed to discover dysponetic functioning in specific systems and then help people to adjust the faulty functioning before it develops into a chronic symptom or severe disorder. Using muscle electro-myographic (EMG) feedback, for example, Kohli and Whatmore have treated patients with digestive–system disturbance, depression, eczema, and neurodermatitis.

Muscle feedback has been used successfully by Budzynski and Stoyva[13] for systematic desensitization in the treatment of dysponetic, phobic responses. In such work, the person is asked to imagine a troubling scene. As the tension level increases, the EMG signals increase, indicating stress. When the stress level becomes excessive, he or she gradually relaxes and lets the fear–provoking scene dissolve until the low EMG level has been reached. Once the scene is thought of again, repetition of the process can again eliminate unwanted high–arousal effects. In this way, biofeedback helps one to "desensitize" oneself and slough off an undesirable stress reaction.

Electromyographic feedback and relaxation has been used to wean individuals from their tranquilizers and soporifics. A combination of EMG feedback and breathing techniques is used to help patients who respond to stress by using tranquilizers and sleeping pills, to become more resilient and more relaxed at their offices and in their homes.[14–20]

Unstressing through biofeedback therapy has also been successful in the amelioration of hypertension. Moeller and Love[14] used EMG feedback from the frontalis muscle group of the forehead combined with autogenic homework exercises to teach nine hypertensive patients to enter into and maintain deeply relaxed states. These patients were given one–half hour of biofeedback once a week for 17 weeks. They achieved an average of 15 percent decrease in both systolic and diastolic pressure after training. Electromyographic feedback has also been used to induce a specific relaxation response in the treatment of migraine, tension headaches, ulcerative proctitis, and spastic colon disorders which are the result of "fight or flight" stress reactions no longer either appropriate or useful.

Biofeedback for neuromuscular rehabilitation is an area of considerable importance. It is a very efficient method for helping individuals regain control over their bodies following a period of paralysis due to a stroke or accident. Johnson and Garton[15] have had encouraging results with ten hemiplegic patients, all but one of whom had been paralyzed for at least a year. Marinacci,[16] a researcher in electromyography, has had success treating partial paralysis due to stroke and has used EMG feedback with some success in cases of Bell's palsy, causalgia, nerve injury, and residual anterior poliomyelitis. Booker and his colleagues[17] have successfully retrained the facial muscle of a patient following spinal accessory–facial–nerve anastomosis. Though these results are remarkable, there is one limitation of EMG feedback in neuromuscular rehabilitation: therapy must be started quite soon after the injury, before bad habits have formed or there is musucular atrophy.

Disorders of the cardiovascular system have been treated effectively with biofeedback through direct monitoring of blood pressure and heart rate. Biofeedback techniques whose primary aim is the attainment of deeply relaxed states elicit a generalized relaxation response which can also aid in the treatment of cardiovascular, particularly hypertension. In one early study, Benson, Shapiro, Tursky, and Schwartz[18] used biofeedback to obtain significant decreases in systolic blood pressures in patients with hypertension. However, no attempt was made to introduce the laboratory–designed exercises into the patient's daily lives or to evaluate the persistence of lowered pressure outside the laboratory.

More recently, Gary E. Schwartz, of Yale University, has taught individuals to regulate several cardiovascular functions simultaneously. Schwartz[19] focused his research design on what he calls "patterns of physiological responses in the generation of subjective experience." This research is one of the most convincing and remarkable demonstrations of the specificity of human self–regulation.

With his colleagues, David Shapiro and Bernard Turksy, Schwartz began a series of experiments on systolic blood pressure and heart rate. Subjects in the experiment were given audio feedback indicating the regulation of one of four possible states: blood pressure up and heart rate up; blood pressure up and heart rate down; blood pressure down and heart rate up; and blood pressure down, heart rate down. Initially, it was found that individuals could learn to regulate their blood pressure in a single session and that these changes were independent of heart rate. In fact, it appeared that systolic blood pressure and heart rate were related in a random manner.

One question which arose was whether or not a person could learn to control both processes simultaneously. In order to resolve this issue, subjects were given feedback only when a desired pattern occurred. When the subjects were required to produce an integrated pattern of either blood pressure and heart rate up or blood pressure and heart rate down, they showed simultaneous control of both functions in the same direction. This was in direct contrast to the previous findings which showed that specific control over either heart rate or blood pressure did not necessarily induce a simultaneous change in the other function. More importantly yet, the feedback for these integrated patterns produced more rapid learning and somewhat larger changes than the feedback for the single function.

Perhaps the most significant conclusion drawn from the observation that blood pressure and heart rate did not vary together is that it is possible for an individual to fragment the functions of his neurophysiological system, and create a disruptive pattern. This fragmentation can occur entirely without the person's awareness. It may be that these splits occur more frequently than current practitioners recognize and that discontinuities between psychological and physiological processes constitute the essence of psychosomatic disorders.[20–21] If such fragmentations a harmonious intelead to dysfunction, a harmonious integration of mind and body functions and restoration of integrated physiological response could be an important goal of health maintenance.

While many research and clinical applications of biofeedback, such as thermal feedback for vascular migraine are quite developed, there are innovative areas at the frontiers of clinical biofeedback. Among these is regulation of highly specific biological functions with increasingly precise sensors. Here the emphasis is placed on developing the proper sensors for the specific functions to be regulated.

One such application involves the use of a small strain gauge around the penile shaft giving feedback about the degree of penile erection to men trying to overcome impotence.[22] Another innovative biofeedback system has been developed by Paul Gorman and Joe Kamiya,[23] who have been teaching individuals to regulate their stomach acidity,—a first step toward a therapeutic program for ulcers. In other research laboratories, air–resistance feedback has been used to teach individuals to recognize changes in their bronchial tube diameter, a measurement that may have significance for the treatment of asthma and other respiratory disease.[24] Other experimental uses of biofeedback include electroocculographic or EOG feedback, which involves the feeding back of muscle tension around the eyes for the correction of visual disorders ranging from near– and farsightedness to glaucoma.[25] Auditory feedback from the small intestine helps sufferers of chronic diarrhea or chronic constipation.[26] Regulation of epileptic seizure activity has sometimes occurred through EEG biofeedback.

The research on seizures is particularly suggestive. It was inititated by M. Barry Sterman, of the Veterans' Hospital in Sepulveda, California. Sterman, beginning his research with cats, noted a discrete 12–16–Hz rhythm over their sensorimotor cortex when the cats remained immobile. Since this frequency was characteristic of immobility and since epilepsy can be considered as hypermobility, he concluded that the deliberate induction of 12–16–cycle activity might be a means of eliminating seizure activity. Sterman trained four psychomotor epileptics to produce this brainwave activity, which he termed the "sensorimotory rhythm" or SMR. Using biofeedback over a six–to–eight–month period they were able to produce a significant decrease in seizure activity.[27–28]

Control of a chronic pain symptom notoriously susceptible to psychological influence is another medical problem to which biofeedback has been applied. Alpha feedback has been used to aid in the overcoming of intractable pain due to postoperative or phantom–limb syndromes. An abundance of alpha activity appears to help an individual remove himself psychologically from the pain so as not to react to it as intensely. Patients still feel the pain, but it is usually reported as a dull sensation rather than a sharp or throbbing one.[29]

Biofeedback has a range of other health promotion and disease prevention possibilities. It can be used to train people to enter hypo–aroused states, which are characterized by theta or very low EMG levels. These meditative states are claimed by some to be ideal for self–programming and sleep–learning.[30] While in these states people can interrogate their "unconscious" to obtain information concerning a pressing problem before it leads to excessive anxiety or physical symptoms. Elmer E. and Alyce Green[31] have been using theta–feedback training to develop their subjects' capacity for imagery, creativity, and integrative experiences. The Greens feel that theta activity is a threshold between the conscious and the unconscious, a state in which a person can achieve subtle levels of psychological and physiological awareness. From their experience in this state these individuals gain a profound sense of trust in their own inner experience and feel more free to allow their creativity to unfold.

Future biofeedback uses could range from this kind of consciousness expansion to even more sophisticated clinical uses: vaginal feedback systems to control fertility and yeast infections; thermographic photography to help a woman regulate the temperature and blood in the area of a breast tumor. If a patient can increase the hypothermic activity in the region of the tumor then perhaps she can starve the tumor of nutrients by shutting down its blood supply; on the other hand, increasing blood flow in the area may enhance the local immunological competence and thereby curtail the tumor. In either case, biofeedback raises the possibility of nonsurgical intervention with breast tumors.

Many of the biological sensors mentioned here are experimental and not available for clinical applications at the present time. Innovations in biomedical technology are making new biofeedback instrumentation widely available within a matter of a few years. Each innovative application should, however, be carefully assessed and developed prior to its application in clinical settings. And all use of biofeedback technology should be accompanied by the warning that no degree of biomedical sophistication should blind us to the requirements of an individual person; such instrumentation ultimately involves the cooperation of the patient.

Toward Mind–Body Integration and Self–Control

Since psychophysiological functions may not necessarily be linked together, it is possible for individuals to fraction or fragment their neurophysiological systems into a disruptive pattern. Indeed a neurophysiological dysfunction can occur without an individual's awareness. The relaxation response, a state of mind–body integration in which emotional and physiological calm prevails, represents the antithesis of this disruptive pattern. Through a comprehensive diagnostic system in clinical biofeedback, various kinds of psychosomatic fragmentations can be classifed. Once a fragmented, dysfunctional pattern has been identified, a general relaxation procedure—induced through clinical biofeedback or meditative techniques may be combined with techniques designed to bring about the regulation of the particular dysfunctional system or organ.

In its most fundamental terms, the principle underlying a holistic approach to clinical biofeedback is that the whole person can be qualitatively different from the sum of his or her parts and yet be dependent upon the organization of these parts for a unique state of psychosomatic integration and health. The future directions of clinical biofeedback should not lead to the indiscriminate application of biomedical instrumentation but to increasingly sensitive holistic adaptations for each individual. Thus the frontiers will be expanded not only by current technology but by the creativity of researchers and clinicians in shaping a health–care system in which the patient's dignity, self–regulation, and growth are enhanced and developed.

Quite often, voluntary regulation of internal states enables patients to alleviate the symptoms of their psychogenic disorder through their own efforts, without external intervention in the form of medications or surgery. While voluntary control of internal states has only just begun to be applied to the prevention and treatment of disease, already it has become a potentially revolutionary force in the future o: preventive health care. Techniques of self–regulation have the effect of returning to the individual a sense of efficacy and control over his or her own life and health—the loss of which can be an insidious effect of excessive stress. The helplessness and hopelessness that may accompany chronic stress weaken psychological resistance and immunological response. Individuals may begin their recovery by realizing that self–regulation can extend to all areas of their life, giving them power to orient their lifestyle in a more positive direction. Biofeedback is a tool for altering psychology as well as physiology.

Learning to control a basic, biological function such as peripheral circulation or muscle activity allows patients to directly experience the interaction between mind and body as well as their own capacity to affect it both positively and negatively. Thus realizing they can have some effect upon the course and alleviation of their disorders, they are no longer passive victims. In the strength of this knowledge patients become active participants with their doctors in alleviating their condition and preventing further occurrences.

Just as psychogenic factors play a considerable part in the etiology and duration of illness, so they may profoundly influence healing and sometimes swing the balance between life and death. Arnold A. Hutschnecker's book, *The Will to Live,* and the visualization methods of radiologist O. Carl Simonton and other clinicians treating cancer patients, underscore the vital part that an individual's will can play in the outcome of any disease.[21,32] Indeed, patients may emerge from an illness with increased rather than impaired functioning. The relationship between the psychological predisposition of the individual to recover and its effect upon actual recovery must continue to be explored.

At the same time that researchers and clinicians strive toward stress alleviation, it is of utmost importance to remember that not all stress can or should be eliminated. An elevated level of neurophysiological activity during exercise or transient crisis is not synonymous with chronic, unabated stress. Individual development requires a variety of kinds of stimulation, and a sedentary, carefree lifestyle does not mean health. Periods of illness, stress, or crisis in a perons's life can be a time of profound personal transformation. Such occurrences offer an individual and those about him the opportunity for major life changes. In a very real sense, a breakdown can be a breakthrough.[33-34]

We must remember that physical and psychological illness are potentially regenerative rather than inherently degenerative. Illness can be a period of time to reexamine fundamental values and priorities, a productive rather than a destructive period of time. In his early writings, C. G. Jung noted that primitive people interpreted illness not as a weakness of the conscious mind but rather as evidence of the inordinate strength of the unconscious mind as it transforms an individual from one stage of life to another. In this context symptoms may be an indication of an individual's attempt to undergo a profound self–healing process, a process which may be disrupted, rather than enhanced, by excessive medication. Reduction of the excessive and potentially lethal aspects of this transition may be desirable, but this does not mean reducing the individual to a state of complacent lethargy.

A holistic approach, integrating techniques ranging from ancient meditative systems to twentieth–century biomedical technology must, however, always emphasize individuals' capacity for self–control and growth, their ability to strive for, and maintain themselves in harmony with their environment.

References

1. Selye, H. *The stress of life.* New York: McGraw Hill, 1956.
2. Dubos, R. *Man adapting.* New Haven: Yale University Press, 1965.
3. Holmes, T. H., & Rahe, R. H. The social readjustment rating scale. *Journal of Psychosomatic Research*, 1967, *11*, 213–218.
4. Wintrobe, M. M., Thora, G. W., Adams, R. A., Brauawald, E., Isselbecker, K.J., Petersdorf, R. A. *Harrison's principles of internal medicine.* New York: McGraw Hill, 1972.
5. Simeons, A. T. W. *Man's presumptuous brain: An evolutionary interpretation of psychosomatic disease.* New York: Dutton, 1961.
6. Bateson, G. *Steps to an ecology of mind.* New York: Ballantine Books, 1972.
7. Friedman, M., & Rosenman, R. H. *Type A behavior and your heart.* New York: Knopf, 1974.
8. Le Shan, L. A basic psychological orientation apparently associated with malignant disease. *The Psychiatric Quarterly*, 1911, 36,37: 314–330.
9. Kissen, D. M. The significance of personality in lung cancer. *Psychophysiological Aspects of Cancer.* E. M. Meyer & H. Hutchins (Eds.), New York: New York Academy of Sciences, 1966, pp. 933–945.
10. Blackwell, B. Minor tranquilizers: Misuse or overuse? *Psychosomatics*, 1975, *16*, 28–31.
11. Green, E. D., Green, A. M., & Walters, E. D. Voluntary control of internal states: Psychological and physiological. *Journal of Transpersonal Psychology*, 1970, *2*, 1–26.

12. Whatmore, G.B., & D. R. Hohli. Dysponesis: A neurophysiologic factor in functional disorders. *Behavioral Science*, 1968, *13*, 102–24.

13. Budzynski, T. H., J. M. Stoyva and C. Adler, "Feedback induced muscle relaxation: application to tension headache. *J. of Behavior Therapy and Experimental Psychiatry*, I, 1970; 205–211.

14. Moeller, T. A., Love, W. A. Jr. A method to reduce arterial hypertention through muscular relaxation. Paper presented at the Biofeedback Research Society Meeting, Boston, 1972.

15. Johnson, H. E. & Garton, W. H. *A practical method of muscle reeducation in hemiplegia: Electromyographic facilitation and conditioning.* Unpublished manuscript, Casa Colina Hospital, Pomona, California, 1973.

16. Marinacci, A. A. *Applied electromyography.* Philadelphia: Lea and Febiger, 1968.

17. Booker, H. E., Rubow, R. T. & Coleman, P. J. Simplified feedback in neuromuscular retraining: An automated approach using electromyographic signals. *Archives of Physical Medicine and Rehabilitation, IV*, 1969, 615–621.

18. Benson, H., Shapiro, D., Tursky, B., & Schwartz, G. E. Decreased systolic blood pressure through operant conditioning techniques in patients with essential hypertension. *Science*, 1971, 173–740.

19. Schwartz, G. E. "Disregulation and systems theory: A biobehavioral framework for biofeedback and behavioral medicine," in Shapiro, D., Stoyva, J., Kaniya, J. Barber, T. X., Miller N. E. and Schwaltz, G. R. (Eds). *Biofeedback and Behavioral Medicine (1979-80)* NY, Aldine, 1981. pp. 27–59.

20. Pelletier, K. R., Peper, E. The Chutzpah Factor in the Psychophysiology of altered states of consciousness. in G. Hendricks & J. Fadiman (Eds.). *Transpersonal education: A curriculum for feeling and being.* New York: Prentice–Hall, 1976.

21. Pelletier, K. R. *Holistic Medicine.* New York: Delacorte, 1979.

22. Eversaul, G. Psychophysiology training and the behavioral treatment of premature ejaculation: Preliminary findings. *Proceedings of the Biofeedback Research Society.* Denver: Biofeedback Research Society, 1975.

23. Gorman, P., & Kamiya, J. Voluntary control of stomach pH. Research note presented at the Biofeedback Research Society Meeting, Boston, November, 1972.

24. Vachon, L. *Biofeedback in action, Medical World News,* March 9, 1973.

25. Sanella, L. "Biofeedback and glaucoma" Paper presented at Kaiser Permanente Hospital, Oakland, California—Dept. of Opthamology, 1979.

26. Stroebel, C. Personal Communication, 1975.

27. Sterman, M. B. Neurophysiological and clinical studies of sensorimotor EEG biofeedback training: Some effects on epilepsy, in L. Birk (Ed.), *Seminars in Psychiatry.* New York: Grune and Stratton, 1974, *5*, 507–525.

28. Sterman, M. B. Clinical implications of EEG biofeedback training: A critical appraisal, in G. E. Schwartz & J. Beatty, (Eds.) *Biofeedback: Theory and Research*. New York: Academic Press, 1975, Chapter 18.

29. Pelletier, K. R. & Peper, E. Developing a biofeedback model: Alpha EEG feedback as a means for pain control, *Biofeedback and Self–Regulation*. In press, 1977.

30. Budzynski, T. H., & Peffer, K. Twilight state learning: The presentation of learning material during a biofeedback–produced altered state. *Proceedings of the Biofeedback Research Society*. Denver: Biofeedback Research Society., 1974.

31. Green, E. E., Green, A. M., and Walters, E. D. "Voluntary control of internal states: psychological and physiological." *J of Transpersonal Psychology* 2, (1970): 1-26.

32. Simonton, O. C., Simonton, S. Belief systems and mangement of the emotional aspects of malignancy, *Journal of Transpersonal Psychology*, 1975, 7(1), 29–48.

33. Laing, R. D. *The politics of experience*. New York: Ballantine Books, 1969.

34. Perry, J. W. The reconstitutive process in the psychopathology of the self. *Annals of the New York Academy of Science*, 1962, *96*, 853–876.

Part III

WORKING WITH THE BODY

Modern physicians have tended at times to neglect truths that were obvious to our ancestors. Touch and right nutrition, for example, are profoundly important parts of all healing traditions. No less an authority than Hippocrates urged his followers to "let food be your medicine and medicine your food." And acupuncture, largely misunderstood or ignored in the West, has been the centerpiece of Chinese health care for several millennia. The essays in this section offer clinical and research evidence which suggests that we often neglect these important domains of health care.

The section begins with Chapter 6 by Robert Rodale, consumer health advocate, and publisher of *Prevention* magazine. Rodale marshalls evidence to demonstrate that by violating the "historical program" of our ancestors' diets, we have endangered our health.

Robert Rodale is the Editor of *Organic Gardening, New Farm, New Shelter,* and *Prevention* magazines. He is chairman of the board and chief executive officer of Rodale Press, Inc., and president of the Soil and Health Foundation, Emmaus, Pennsylvania. Mr. Rodale has written and lectured extensively on nutrition and preventive medicine, and has authored *The Basic Book of Organic Gardening* (Ballantine, 1970), *Sane Living in a Mad World* (Rodale, 1972), and *The Best Health Ideas I Know* (Rodale, 1974).

Chapters 7 and 8 by Drs. Robert Swearingen and Dolores Krieger focus on the importance of touch. Swearingen, an orthopedist, describes the rediscovery of his own body—hands and heart as well as head—as a therapeutic instrument.

Dr. Robert L. Swearingen is clinical instructor, Department of Orthopedic Surgery, University of Colorado School of Medicine, director of the Summit Center in Frisco, Colorado, and a member of the American Academy of Orthopedic Surgeons. As an orthopedist practicing in both a large ski area and in a suburban community, his experiences range from emergency room techniques designed to decrease the amount of pain medication needed to attempts to hasten bone healing by meditation and visualization.

Dolores Krieger, R.N., Ph.D., outlines the scientific evidence for a healing force that is not yet physically detectable. She describes "therapeutic touch," a hands–on technique communicating this healing force from practitioner to patient, documenting it with carefully controlled studies revealing its profound physiological effects.

Dr. Krieger is a professor of nursing, New York University School of Education, Health, and Nursing and the Art Professions, Division of Nursing, New York City; member of Sigma Pheta Tau; and New York Regional and National consultant on Spinal Cord Injuries to the

Veterans Administration, Washington, D.C. She has developed at New York University the first university–based course at the Masters level on healing by human field interaction.

The section concludes with Chapter 9, an overview of the therapeutic utility of acupuncture by Drs. Michael Volen, and David Bresler, clinicians who have successfully applied therapeutic touch in their work at UCLA Pain Control Unit and in private practice.

Michael P. Volen, M.D., is the former clinical medical director of the UCLA Pain Control Unit and Associate Physician in the Department of Anesthesiology, UCLA School of Medicine. He is the author of numerous publications on acupuncture, nutrition, and pain control and is now in private practice in Arcata, California.

Chapter 6

NUTRITION:
THE HISTORICAL IMPERATIVE

Robert Rodale

Human life has existed for at least five million years. During that long period of time, the appearance and inner workings of the human organism have gradually evolved in response to environmental conditions. But that process of change was extremely slow, and as far as we know there have been no significant changes in our physical make-up in at least 40,000 years.

"The evolution of Homo sapiens had been essentially completed some 100,000 years ago," Rene Dubos[1] has said. "In other words, mankind has retained the same fundamental characteristics, potentialities, and limitations since the late Paleolithic period, when the genetic code of Homo sapiens achieved its present formula."

Dubos continues by warning that there is no chance that this genetic endowment can be safely or usefully modified in the foreseeable future. Biological limitations on Homo sapiens condition the extent to which lifestyles and the environment can be changed by technology.

What were the prehistoric environmental conditions which forged these biological limitations? There was, in fact, no agriculture at all during the major part of our period of evolutionary development— modern crops like corn, wheat and rice were not available. People ate

89

the flesh of fish and wild animals. Seeds, stems, roots, and fruit of wild plants and even so-called weeds were eaten in great quantities. Whole categories of food which are now eaten in large amounts were hardly available at all during early human history. Sugar, for example, now eaten at every meal by a majority of people was a rare treat prior to the modern age, available only in certain seasons in the form of ripe fruits or the honey of wild bees.

Salt, also, during the long range of human history, was usually hard to get. Sometimes people suffered from salt deficiencies. Our bodies have been shaped by this low–salt environment, tuned to achieve maximum health on an intake of about 500 milligrams a day. Currently, however, people in the United States consume an average of ten grams of salt a day.

Animal fat has changed in both quality and amount in the diet since precivilized times. A wild pig has much less fat on its carcass than a modern, domesticated pig. The nature of that fat has changed, to a large degree, also, from unsaturated to saturated. "In effect the balance between nonessential and essential animal fats is 50 to one in the domestic animal and about two to one in the free living animal," state Michael and Sheilagh Crawford in their book, *What We Eat Today*.[2] The effects of such changes in the basic composition and amounts of fat in the diet are apparent in the people who eat those foods and from what we know of their health problems: They are overweight and have fat–related disorders.

Fiber in food is also an important factor in our evolutionary history. Our ancient diet patterns included many high–fiber, unrefined foods. For that reason, the human gut is tuned to function most effectively only when a suitable amount of fiber is present in foods. The diet of highly refined cereals and other carbohydrates typical of people living in industrialized societies is lacking in sufficient fiber, and is a cause of some important health problems.

DIETARY CHANGES AND THEIR CONSEQUENCES

Anyone who reads the medical and health literature regularly will see occasional references to "man's evolutionary history" in discussions of reasons for the existence of a particular disease or nutritional problem. Where we have come from in our long–range history is extremely important to our current welfare; there is no easy way for us to escape the bounds of our evolutionary history. These facts, recognized by researchers, have yet to be construed as a tool for analyzing the value of health and research goals or, more importantly, for planning effective systems of health improvement.

In order to do that, I have given the name "inner historical program" to the unchangeable facets of human nature impressed upon us by our evolutionary history. This phrase indicates that we are programmed internally in the same fashion as a computer, but the software in this case is an evolutionary history that cannot be changed. By ignoring the dictates of this program and continuing to eat foods incompatible with this program for a certain period of time, we may soon face serious and perhaps irreversible problems.

Consider the case of sugar. It is estimated that each American consumes close to 138 pounds of sugar a year. Even more alarming, three–quarters of this sugar intake is "invisibly" consumed as an ingredient of the foods we buy in modern supermarkets. The presence of sugar in processed and convenience foods is so all–pervasive that it is difficult to choose randomly a supermarket food item that does not contain added sugar in some form.

Despite its liberal use, the nutritional fact remains that we do not need refined sugar products at all. Our bodies do need certain sugars for energy, but over the course of man's evolutionary history, those natural sugars have been obtained very nicely from vegetables, cereal grains, and fruits. The human digestive system has been programmed in such a way that we can convert the starch in vegetables to sugars to give us all the energy we need.

As John Yudkin, a British physician and biochemist, points out,[3] fairly recently in terms of man's evolutionary span—about 2,500 years ago—that man first learned to produce a crude, concentrated sort of sugar by extracting and drying the sap of the sugar cane. Although cultivation of sugar cane gradually spread—to China, the Mediterranean, Arabia, Brazil, and other areas—the cost of sugar remained prohibitively high.

Only as a result of the development of sugar plantations in the Caribbean, based on slave labor, did the modern sugar industry come into being. Since the middle of the eighteenth century, the increased demand combined with technological advances in growing, extracting, and refining sugar drove prices down. Thus consumption of sugar has risen to the exceedingly high levels of today.

What are some of the health consequences of this rapid dietary shift? The demonstrable medical fact is that sugar's first target is the teeth. Yudkin[4] has noted that in his studies of dental caries in 15 to 18 year olds, a positive correlation existed between the degree of dental caries and the amount of sugar taken in solid foods. We know that when table sugar is introduced into cultures which have never known this "luxury," dental problems soon appear. On the other hand, primitive people who have not been exposed to sugar have few, if any, cavities.

In one way or another, excess sugar consumption has been associated with most of the degenerative diseases that strike modern humans, including obesity, heart disease, and diabetes. If we compute our average annual sugar consumption at 138 pounds per person, we are each receiving approximately 660 "empty" calories a day—the energy equivalent of 69 pounds of flab per year.

Obesity is one direct consequence of our sugar–rich society. Conservative estimates indicate that 10 to 20 percent of all U.S. children and 20 to 25 percent of all middle–aged Americans are overweight. Other nutrition writers, including Yudkin, speculate that a high–sugar diet contributes the the rising incidence of diabetes by driving the pancreas to exhaustion in its attempts to produce enough insulin to maintain proper blood–sugar (glucose) levels.

Too much sugar in the diet can override the body's inner historical program in another way: by causing hypoglycemia, a condition in which the body's circulating supply of energy–giving glucose dips abnormally. Too many candy bars, soft drinks, or other refined carbohydrates can cause the body's glucose–regulating mechanism to overreact—thus bringing on hypoglycemia.

Because glucose is the only "fuel" it can burn, the brain is particularly sensitive to severe fluctuations in circulating blood sugar. As a result, hypoglycemic individuals often complain of dizziness, tremor, fainting, headaches, fatigue, sweating, or other vague symptoms a few hours after eating high–sugar snacks.

According to Jose A. Yaryura–Tobias of Bio–behavioral Psychiatry in Great Neck, New York, violations of the inner historical program—from eating too much spaghetti, pizza, cake, white bread, alcohol, and other staples of the American diet—can trigger uncontrollably violent behavior in certain individuals. "It is our feeling that there are numerous people suffering from this condition," he says.

For more than five years, drawing from the clinical experience of more than 70 patients, Dr. Yaryura–Tobias and his colleagues have been studying the link between violent behavior and impaired glucose metabolism. "Patients present a long–standing history of aggressive behavior, many times since childhood," Dr. Yaryura–Tobias reports. "Every person does have a normal amount of violent thought, but in these patients, the amount of violent thought is excessive and may interfere with normal thought processes."

Good results have been achieved by putting these people on an antihypoglycemic diet designed to smooth out the intake of food energy over the course of the day. Foods with moderate–to–high quantities of protein, fat, and fiber are favored because, unlike sugar and other refined carbohydrates, they tend to be digested slowly, keeping blood sugar on an even keel.

Excess salt provides another striking illustration of dietary deviation from the inner historical program leading to serious health consequences. Because of the scarcity of salt in the environment, our human system developed and evolved to need less than one twenty–fifth of an ounce daily—without which the body automatically excretes fluids to keep the inner salt content in balance. As civilization advanced, however, and people began using salt to preserve meat and to pickle and ferment vegetables for storage, the average salt intake increased far beyond our actual requirement. Common daily intakes in America range from seven to 15 grams per person, with many individuals consuming as much as 30 grams per day. Even the suggested requirement of five grams represents as much as 10 times the amount on which adequate sodium balance can be maintained.

Why is so much salt used? There are two reasons. The first and more obvious one is that salting food heavily is a cultural addiction. Many people have become adjusted to the taste of salt in food and drinks, having acquired that taste addiction as tiny babies, from processed infant food salted to taste good to mothers.

The second reason is that salt is part of almost every processed food. Sardines, mustard, soup, bread and olives all contain salt, as does cheese, processed meat, soy sauce, and just about every other packaged food. Trying to cut down of salt while still eating processed foods is a difficult task.

When we eat a lot of salt, the amount of fluid retained between the cells is increased. Large amounts of this extracellular fluid force the heart to work harder pushing blood through the kidney's filtering system. This effort can result in essential hypertension or high blood pressure, one of the most serious health problems of this age.

The connection between salt use and high blood pressure has been suspected for over 70 years. In recent years, evidence implicating salt has accumulated from so many sources that an almost overwhelming case for the salt–hypertension correlation has been made.

Studies of the salt–use habits of primitive tribes have revealed that primitive people with access to salt who use it as a condiment and food preservative have problems with high blood pressure. Those people who still live the way people have been conditioned to live by their inner historical programs—that is, with only tiny amounts of salt—have almost no high blood pressure.

In an extremely useful article on salt and hypertension, Edward D. Freis[5] describes some striking cross–cultural findings. For example, F. W. Lowenstein went into the Brazilian jungle and looked at the health of two tribes living near each other. People in the Mundurucus tribe, converted to Christianity by missionaries and introduced to salt, though very primitive in other respects, typically had high blood pressure which tended to rise as they got older. The nearby Carajos tribe, with no contact at all with Western civilization and who used no table salt had no hypertension at all. According to Freis and others, similar correlations between salt use, colonization, and hypertension have been found among inhabitants of the Solomon Islands, New Guinea, Malaysia, Ugunda, and the Kalahari Desert of Africa.

Dr. Freis points out that people must reduce their salt intake to about one gram "to produce more than a minimal reduction of blood pressure." This is possible to do if one stays away from all processed foods and avoids using the salt shaker. Despite small amounts of salt occurring naturally in meat, eggs, and even vegetables, a diet of unsalted fresh meats, eggs, vegetables, and grains can keep within that one–gram (1,000 mg.) level. But making exceptions for processed foods quickly puts one over the limit.

Excess salt has also been found to trigger attacks of Meniere's disease, a disturbance of the inner ear which causes thousands of Americans to suffer a sensation comparable in severity and quality to certain forms of seasickness. Under medical management a majority of Meniere's victims can be satisfactorily controlled on a strict low–salt diet. Roger Boles of the University of California[6] reported that 63 of 103 patients with severe Meniere's disease had no episodes of dizziness following salt restriction. Another 26 had a good response, reducing the severity and number of attacks to only one in three months.

Whereas problems have arisen from too much salt and sugar in the modern food supply, a third substance, fiber, is now in critically short supply. As Denis P. Burkitt[7] has pointed out, the amount of natural food fiber in the Western diet plummeted by more than 90 percent in the period between 1880 and 1960, largely as a result of new grain refining techniques. The loss of this nonnutritive bulk, to which the human gut had become adapted over history, has had deleterious consequences. According to Neil S. Painter[8–9] of the Manor House Hospital, London, the normal functioning of the intestinal tract depends upon the presence of adequate fiber which absorbs water and forms soft bulk. When deprived of fiber—as in the typical American diet of white flour, sugar, meat, and dairy foods—the gut performs abnormally.

One consequence may be diverticulosis, a disease characterized by small pouches in the colon wall caused by the enormous pressure needed for propelling small, hard stools. About 70 percent of all westerners over age 70 show some signs of this disease, which can be extremely painful if the sacs become inflamed. Yet, as Dr. Painter points out, fewer than ten cases have been observed in rural Africa in the last 12 years, presumably because rural Africans eat a diet high in fiber, including potatoes, beans, bananas, and unrefined cornmeal. The large, moist stools formed by this regimen keeps the bowels in good working order. It's important to note, though, that when Africans forsake their historical diet and begin to eat a "civilized" low–fiber diet, they also get diverticulosis.

In another study, by Brodribb and Humphreys[10] at the Royal Berkshire Hospital in Reading, England, every one of 40 patients with diverticulosis who was fed bran improved. Sixty percent of all symptoms—from bloody stools, distension, and pain to flatulence and wind—were totally eliminated. This kind of information had led researchers to speculate that bran and other natural dietary fiber act as bowel normalizers, relieving both constipation and diarrhea, and speeding up overly slow intestinal transit times.

By serving as an obstacle to caloric intake, fiber may also help to prevent obesity. K.W. Heaton[11] of the Bristol Royal Infirmary has noted that people eating whole wheat bread tend to excrete about three times as many calories a day as they do when they eat the same amount of white bread. In addition, high–fiber foods utilize total capacity to chew and digest, distending the stomach and creating a satisfied, "full" feeling that helps prevent overeating.

THE CONTENT AND PREPARATION OF MEALS

Cooking has become almost an obsession. As a result, some of us may go days, weeks, or months without eating anything that hasn't been cooked. So far as we are able to tell, this may be inimical to good health.

For example, John M. Douglass, an internist at the Southern California Permanente Medical Group, Los Angeles, has been using a raw–food diet to treat his diabetic patients. The majority of those who have followed this diet have been able to reduce their insulin requirement. Dr. Douglass reported that one patient had his insulin requirement reduced from 60 to 15 units per day solely by dietary management, and another had his insulin requirement reduced from 70 units per day to diet control alone.[12,13] Both of these changes were accomplished by increasing the percentage of raw food in their diets.

The rationale for prescribing a raw–food diet is based on Dr. Douglass' belief that early man lived entirely on raw food and that such a diet would be less stressful to the human system and less likely to produce diabetes than a cooked–food diet. Why the diet is effective is not known, but according to Dr. Douglass, "It may have to do with the interaction of the noninactivated enzymes that are present in raw items or with the fast transit time that is inherent in a raw diet.[11] In his most recent work, Dr. Douglass has stated that raw–food diets can help lower high blood pressure and reduce overweight.

One simple way to increase the quantity and quality of raw food in the American diet would be for more people to eat freshly sprouted seeds and beans. Sprouting not only increases the protein quality of those foods, it boosts vitamin values as well. Soybeans, for instance, contain 12 times the vitamin C content when in the form of sprouts. In peas, the increase is from zero to 38 milligrams of vitamin C per three and one-half ounces after only four days of sprouting. Riboflavin (B_2) increases 13 times when oats are sprouted; the folic acid content of wheat quadruples. It seems then that by digging up and eating the first succulent green sprouts and shoots of spring, our primitive ancestors were demonstrating an unconscious nutritional wisdom.

More dietary emphasis on natural, unprocessed foods—whether raw or cooked—would also help to avoid a peculiarly modern danger: food additives. There is increasing evidence that our metabolic apparatus is not meant to handle many of these very recent additions to the food supply. For example, Reif–Lehrer and Stemmermann[14] have described episodes of shuddering, migranelike seizures and shivering which they traced to monosodium glutamate (MSG) ingestion. They believe that similar MSG–induced problems in youngsters occur with unsuspected frequency. The two researchers point out that MSG: (1) used as a flavor enhancer is a known exciter of neurons, (2) has caused convulsions in animals, and (3) has been linked to brain damage in some animal species. MSG is only one of hundreds of little understood chemicals regularly added to processed foods.

It is ironic that just as we are discovering that many synthetic substances—including many of the drugs prescribed by physicians—may actually be harming the body, we are also rediscovering the primitive wisdom of natural foods as the best medicine. As a final example, a small, but significant minority of the population suffers from an inborn metabolic error that sensitizes them to gluten, the protein portion of grain. For those individuals, eating wheat, rye, barley, buckwheat, or oats can trigger a devastating biological reaction. Symptoms of this condition, known as celiac disease, include severe diarrhea, weight loss, protuberant abdomen, and anemia. Since modern cereal crops, such as wheat, are a relatively recent phenomenon in man's total history, it may be that individuals with celiac disease have in some way been unable to make the biological adjustment to the inner historical program necessary of digesting gluten.

The strong, but baffling association between celiac disease and schizophrenia makes this possibility even more interesting. F. Curtis Dohan[15] of the Eastern Pennsylvania Psychiatric Institute, first suspected such a connection when he observed that certain substances excreted in the urine of schizophrenics were also found in the urine of celiacs.

Dohan's observations of himself and others indicated that celiac disease and schizophrenia occurred in the life of the same individual far more frequently than chance. When Dr. Dohan decided to test gluten sensitivity by introducing a gluten–free diet, he found that, after 110 days, twice as many people on the cereal–free diet were well enough to be discharged as compared with those on a high–cereal diet.

We have an enormous amount of basic research and data–gathering to do before we can piece together all the dietary clues that will help us live in more complete harmony with our inner historical program. But already we know that, along with needed changes in diet, we will also have to adopt other changes in lifestyle if we hope to avoid chronic, degenerative disease at an early age.

LIFESTYLE CHANGES

Physical aspects of modern life other than diet can and do conflict with the inner historical program and should be mentioned here. In prehistoric times, virtually every daily task required the vigorous use of a versatile body. Success meant being able to run fast enough to hunt, to walk far enough to hunt, and to gather nuts and roots, and to strike hard enough to defend against attack. Primitive people who failed those tasks often didn't survive.

The sedentary character of modern life runs directly counter to that physical heritage. Today, most people don't have to work with their muscles to earn a living, so they spend much of their lives in an unnatural state of physical rest and mental tension. They pay the price in a range of illnesses that stem from low–heart–lung fitness and muscular weakness and includes everything from low back pain to certain types of cardiovascular disease.

Even the unnnatural posture of technological life is apparently related to disease. Colin James Alexander[16] has demonstrated a correlation between chair sitting and varicose veins. Eastern and primitive people, who sit on the ground, almost never have varicose veins, whereas people in advanced industrial societies often suffer that affliction.

The chronic, degenerative diseases which result from diets and lifestyles that conflict with the inner historical program have often been called "diseases of civilization." Denis P. Burkitt[7] includes among these conditions "characteristic of modern Western civilization," their "traditional way of life": appendicitis, diverticular disease, benign tumors, cancer of the large bowel, ulcerative colitis, varicose veins, deep vein thrombosis, diabetes, hemorrhoids, coronary heart disease, gall stones, and hiatus hernia.

RESTORING THE INNER HISTORICAL PROGRAM

Prevention is probably the best approach to virtually all health problems, but particularly with degenerative disease which plagues our technological civilization. This does, however, require changes in lifestyle and most particularly diet, which demand considerable effort and motivation.

Implementing prevention on a large scale means educating people to help them preserve the integrity of their primitive inner program in new ways so as not to displace them from our modern, technological society. This large motivational challenge does not itself require a complex technology. Rather, what is required is an eclectic resistance to advanced technology in food, transportation, recreation, and a range of other activities.

A programmatic way to facilitate the dissemination of information about the inner historical program and its imperatives would be to train large numbers of people to act as consulting health educators. In 1969 I outlined the function of consulting health education and suggested areas for training practitioners. Health education is an established profession, but its practitioners concentrate their efforts on children and young people, to whom the question of chronic, degenerative disease is not primarily relevant. Adults receive health information in a fragmented way from a wide variety of sources. However, there is no personal consultant in health education to whom an adult can go seeking answers to important questions about the whole spectrum of health ranging from techniques of exercise to selection of food and avoidance of chemical hazards.

I suggest that doctors give thought to the idea of encouraging the education of men and women to serve as health educators for adults, working in concert with physicians in group practice and on hospital staffs. A descriptive but cumbersome name for this hypothetical new health professional would be "consulting health educator." Perhaps classroom health educators could create a branch of their profession to fulfill the need for direct instruction of adults in effective techniques for selecting and preparing foods, developing exercise regimens and dealing with stress.

The teaching of food and nutrition is usually split into two areas—home economics and experimental nutrition. In few cases is the same person taught in detail both phases of the subject of eating. A consulting health educator should have an understanding not only of the selection, processing, and preparation of food, but of the technical subject of nutrition as well. In that way, he or she might gain new insight into why people eat as they do, what effect the average diet has on health, and how constructive change in diet patterns might be encouraged. This instruction, however, would have to be intensive and comprehensive—not just one or two survey courses.

Consulting health educators would also be trained to counsel people in selecting appropriate forms of ongoing exercise. They would have a good working knowledge of environmental and industrial contaminants, tobacco, and alcohol and their effects on the body. In short, the consulting health educator would be a specialized social worker, a motivator trained to focus on personal health problems and their practical solution. A large part of his or her job would be to help others to live successfully in tune with the inner historical program which we have too long neglected.

REFERENCES

1. Dubos, R. "Adaptation to the Environment and Man's Future," *The Control of the Environment* (J.D. Roslansky, ed.). New York: Fleet Academic Editions, 1971.
2. Crawford, M., and Crawford S. *What We Eat Today: The Food Manipulators vs. the People*. New York: Stein and Day, 1972.

3. Yudkin, J. *Sweet and Dangerous: The New Facts about the Sugar You Eat as a Cause of Heart Disease, Diabetes, and Other Killers.* New York: Peter H. Wyden, 1972.

4. Yudkin, J. "Sugar and Disease." *Nature,* Vol. 239, September 22, 1972, pp. 197–199.

5. Freis, E.D. "Salt Volume and the Prevention of Hypertension," *Circulation,* Vol. 53, No. 4, April, 1976, pp. 589–595.

6. Boles, R., et al. "Conservative Management of Meniere's Disease: Furstenberg Regimen Revisited," *Annals of Otology, Rhinology and Laryngology,* Vol. 84, July-August, 1975, pp. 513–517.

7. Burkitt, D.P. "Some Diseases Characteristic of Modern Western Civilization," *British Medical Journal,* Vol. 1, February 3, 1973, pp. 274–278.

8. Painter, N.S., and Burkitt, D.P., "Diverticular Disease of the Colon: A Deficiency Disease of Western Civilization," *British Medical Journal,* Vol. 2, May 22, 1971, pp. 450–454.

9. Painter, N.S., Almeida, A.Z., and Colebourne, K.W. "Unprocessed Bran in Treatment of Diverticular Disease of the Colon," *British Medical Journal,* Vol. 2, April 15, 1972, pp. 137–140.

10. Brodribb, A.J.M., and Humphreys, D.M. "Diverticular Disease: Three Studies—Part 1—Relation to Other Disorders and Fibre Intake," *British Medical Journal,* Vol. 1, February 21, 1976, pp. 424–430.

11. Heaton, K.W. "Food Fibre as an Obstacle to Energy Intake." *Lancet,* Vol. 2, December 22, 1973, pp. 1418–1421.

12. Douglass, J.M., and Rasgon, I. "Diet and Diabetes," (Letter to editor). *Lancet,* Vol. 2, December 11, 1976, pp. 1306–1307.

13. Douglass, J.M. "Raw Diet and Insulin Requirements," (Letter to editor). *Annals of Internal Medicine,* Vol. 82, No. 1, January, 1975, pp. 61–62.

14. Reif-Lehrer, L., and Stemmermann, M.G. "Monosodium Glutamate Intolerance in Children," (Letter to editor). *New England Journal of Medicine,* Vol. 293, December 4, 1975, p. 1204.

15. Dohan, F.C., and Grasberger, J.C. "Relapsed Schizophrenics: Earlier Discharge from the Hospital After Cereal-Free, Milk-Free Diet." *American Journal of Psychiatry,* Vol. 130, 1973, pp. 685–688.

16. Alexander, C.J. "Chair Sitting and Varicose Veins," *Lancet,* Vol. 1, April 15, 1972, pp. 822–823.

Chapter 7

THE PHYSICIAN AS THE BASIC INSTRUMENT

Robert L. Swearingen, M.D.

As an orthopedist who handles an immense volume of fractures and dislocations in a practice located in one of the largest ski complexes in this country, I have become fascinated with the concept of stress and how it affects the healing process. The search for methods to reduce the effects of stress and to promote the healing process soon began, and an interest in a more holistic approach to medical care naturally follows.

When I think about stress in my patients I usually rate them on a scale of 0 to 100. Each individual has a minute–to–minute average excitation level which is lower in sleep or meditation and higher in periods of external stress or excitation. I have fouind when patients come into the emergency room from the ski slopes their level of excitation will generally indicate both their ability to handle stress and the rate and ease with which their fracture will heal.

If a patient arrives in the emergency room with an injury, say a fracture, and an excitation level of 90, and if that level remains high while we are getting the patient undressed, taking the x–rays, and fixing the injury, then that patient develops a conditioned association between a high excitation level and his fracture. If this happens, every reminder of the fracture—the weight of the cast, and even talking about it during the convalescence—may activate his autonomic nervous system towards the excitation level of 90. This is "hyporest" and is in all probability detrimental to healing.

While in the emergency room I use techniques to lower the excitation level, attempting to couple this injury with a state I consider conducive to body rest and healing. Later I teach the patient methods, which include meditation, to continue the low excitation level throughout convalescence. In this effort I am guided by Benson's work[1] which has shown that the physiological changes in meditation can be considered a form of total rest, and by other research which has indicated that rest is conducive to healing.[2]

Over the years I observed that when I was calm I could easily gain my patient's cooperation. More recently I began to discover that when I was feeling very positive and caring I created an environment around me even more conducive to patient relaxation. I soon learned that my relaxation and caring were contagious: As coworkers began to feel similarly, I observed that they could produce the same effect with patients.

I then began to notice that certain patients who came into the emergency room off the ski slopes appearing much more relaxed than others who were brought in off the ski slopes required less analgesia for the same procedures. I found that these particular patients were always brought in by the same few members of the ski patrol. My staff and I studied the personalities of these patrol persons and in asking them about their approach to patients, found certain common factors. For instance, these ski patrol persons were all genuinely concerned about their patients, approaching them as people first—unlike others who skied up, grabbed the fractured leg, and asked if it hurt. This select group of patrol persons gave permission to their patients to have and express their pain, and intuitively used relaxation techniques.

After studying these common factors, we went to the ski areas and taught entire ski patrols how to adopt a more caring and holistic approach—touching and reassuring, relaxing, and giving permission for the expression of pain while splinting injuries and bringing the person in for care. The great majority of patrol persons could and did use these techniques effectively. The end result was the same as with patrollers who had used such approaches intuitively. The effect in the emergency room was that we were able to decrease the use of pain medication by approximately one–half. Large numbers of our patients began to plan their immediate future with their disability rather than lie around worrying about it.

One particular individual practices this approach with such skill, making such strong contact with patients—thereby relaxing them—that using good stabilization techniques, she can get the ski pants off without cutting a stitch, without analgesics, and without significant pain to the patient. This is medically as well as aesthetically important, for we may need the total safe dose of the analgesic a short time later to set the bones.

HYPERTRACTION AND HEALING

After the patient has been administered to by ski patrol, nurses, and x–ray technicians, he or she is taken to the cast room to have the fracture casted or reduced and then casted. In Summit County we do not have a hospital, and hence we use only intravenous drugs for pain control during reduction (setting and aligning) of fractures. Under such circumstances, I felt that additional traction would not significantly increase the pain to the patient but would enhance the chances of a positive and accurate reduction. One day, after a patient's fractured leg had been flexed at the knee over the side of the cart that he was lying on, I put both my hands around the ankle of the injured leg, then put my legs over my forearms. My assistant was giving countertraction, applying pressure about the patient's knee. The dead weight of my legs resting on my hands applied around 50 pounds of traction, which fatigued the patient's muscles but not mine. Then I hooked my toes under a horizontal shelf on the cart and forcefully but slowly extended my knees, thereby increasing the traction I could apply with my own body.

I found that this procedure consistently improved my reductions. It was especially important for comminuted fractures (in which the bone is broken in several pieces). When we used a scale and compared the amount of traction in the standard method versus what we now call "hypertraction," we were surprised to find that the standard techniques made only 35 percent of the body weight available, whereas hypertraction permitted over 105 percent of the body weight to be applied. For the 175 pound practitioner this represented a threefold increase, from 65 to 185 pounds of traction.

These changes in practitioner behavior provided the basis for a variety of other therapeutic strategies. We focused particularly on the patient's ability to understand the injury and the capacity to influence the recovery process by using relaxation techniques and visualizing rapid healing. Prior to hypertraction I review the x–rays with the patient, explain the fracture, suggest how long it will probably take to heal, describe what type cast will be necessary, and for how long, and explain the procedure I am going to use to put the bone back in place. After the leg has been reduced (or put in a cast if that is all that is necessary), I draw pictures depicting the four stages of the healing process—clot formation around the fracture, the change of the clot into fibrous tissue lattice, calcium crystallization on the latticework, and restructuring of new bone around the fracture site. I explain my concepts of the excitation level and my personal feeling that the healing process can be enhanced by procedures which lower the excitation level and keep it lower (e.g., meditation and visualization).

Most of my patients are just visiting the area where I practice and hence will have their follow-up care elsewhere. Thus I regard it as part of my job to help them find training in meditation and visualization where they live. I let those who do live in my area who wish to use this approach decide whether they want to take a structured course in meditation or to attempt to learn it from a book I recommend; I continue to see them periodically and try to determine whether they are experiencing significant excitation control through meditation; and I help them to use the four drawings of the healing process as a basis for their visualizations. My impression is that since I adopted this approach, the necessary time in the cast and the morbidity during the healing process have both been significantly reduced. At the time of this writing we are developing a research protocol to study and document this process.

WITHOUT MEDICATION AND WITHOUT PAIN

Having worked in major ski areas for nearly 12 years and been faced with up to 80 dislocated shoulders each winter season, I have become interested in the simplest, least invasive, least harmful, and least painful approach to reducing them. In recent years our whole–person approach—talking, touching, making a strong contact with patients, and making them aware of and responsible for their bodies—has made it possible for us to reduce 90 percent of all dislocations without pain medication and without pain.

The evolution of this approach began when I was called to the emergency room to find a young man with a dislocated shoulder lying on the x–ray table. At that time we routinely gave either intravenous medication or full anesthesia for reductions. The reduction was usually associated with quite a bit of pain which was verbally, and freely expressed. I greeted the young man and then went to the x–ray room to verify that the shoulder was indeed dislocated. I returned to the patient and called for the nurse to bring me pain medication. It just so happened that there had been a cardiac arrest and no nurse was available. I sat there looking at the patient and began to sense in myself something akin to panic. It was a feeling of impotence—that without my technological tools I did not feel complete as a physician. I looked at the patient—a man obviously in pain and totally dependent on me— put one hand on the dislocated shoulder in a comforting gesture, and felt his muscles relax. Encouraged by this, I began to talk to him and reassure him. When I explained that we would work together and that I would do nothing without telling him, he relaxed even more. Using the usual manipulative technique I was then able to ease his shoulder back into place without pain medication and without pain.

I am now sure after several years of using and teaching this procedure that all well–trained orthopedists can work with their patients to achieve a low excitation level and that they will be able to reduce virtually all dislocated shoulders in this or a similar manner. My chance of failure, however, is increased if the patient is a fellow physician who feels this approach is not possible and, therefore, cannot relax.

My treatment of these patients was often accompanied by an intuition about which patient was going to do well and which wasn't, which fracture was going to heal rapidly and which was going to heal slowly or even fail to unite. With our responsibility to facilitate healing, if we suspect that someone is going to have difficulty, we should encourage them to learn methods of self-healing. In my experience with stressed individuals, integrative techniques that decrease the excitation level, such as meditation and biofeedback, may be helpful. Other approaches aimed at decreasing the bodily component or manifestation of stress, such as structural integration (Rolfing), bioenergetics, or acupuncture, are also useful in certain circumstances.

More immediately, as physicians we have the power to create either an anxious and stressful environment that inhibits healing or a positive, reassuring atmosphere that can promote it. When a patient with a fractured tibia returns to the orthopedist's office in his first visit since reduction, the complaints of pain are usually minimal compared with the patient's often unspoken need for reassurance. The patient wants to know that he will be able to continue as a meaningful part of society. Though not obvious "physical problems," these are critical needs which we as human beings and physicians can and should address ourselves to.

As physicians and scientists we must also continue to ask ourselves just how meditation, simple reassurance, positive feelings, and visualization can influence the outcome of a fracture. Recent studies[3] on electrical current in the body may provide the beginnings of a scientific answer. Becker has shown that an electrical flow exists at the fracture site and continues until there is either healing or a definitive nonunion. Using small electrodes and a minute current he has been able to stimulate nonunions of many years' duration to heal. It is quite possible that stress and meditation create electrical fields—one which frustrates and the other which promotes healing.

While proceeding with work on the biology of healing and the effects of stress and techniques of stress reduction, we should still remember to ask "Who actually does the healing?" When a patient with a displaced fracture comes in, I align it, cast it, and wait. I wait while the patient heals or does not heal. My responsibility as an orthopedic surgeon is to initiate the healing process with reductions and surgery, to use myself as the basic healing instrument, and then to give the patients tools with which they can heal themselves. A modern version of Pare's classical statement could be, "I treat them and help them heal themselves."

REFERENCES

1. Benson, The Relaxation Response New York: William Morrow, 1975.
2. Ibid
3. Marino, A., Cullen, J., Reichmanis, M. & Becker, R. "Fracture Healing in Rats Exposed to Extremely Low Frequency Electric Fields" *Clinical Orthopedics* 145 pp. 239–244, 1979.

Chapter 8

THERAPEUTIC TOUCH AND THE METAPHYSICS OF NURSING

Dolores Krieger, R.N., Ph.D.

Many of us in the health field have at times been faced with the recognition of inexplicable X factors, the unknowns which appear at variance with everyday reality. A not uncommon occurrence is the client who is apparently recovering but who one day states that he "knows" he is going to die, and, within a few days or even a few hours, does indeed die. Or the patient who seems hopelessly ill, but in spite of our best judgments—and sometimes the patient's own scepticism—goes on to a state of wellness after being "touched" by a person who is known as a "healer" but who may have no formal health–care credentials.

It is only within the last few decades that philosophers of science, such as Northrup[1] and Margenau,[2] have helped us to recognize how rigidly structured are our concepts of the nature of physical reality. Our sense of this reality has been operationally defined: Only if a phenomenon meets particular criteria, measurable in specific terms, do we consider it "real," that is, scientifically acceptable.

These criteria are imposed for good reason—they allow the gradual and painstaking accrual of a common fund of knowledge that is public, replicable, and tolerably firm, but confined. Within these narrow confines we have constructed a world view which may exclude many of the dynamic, energetic, vigorous, and vibrant happenings surrounding us in our daily activities. Now and again hints came to our attention that we have not contained all of reality within our careful definitions. Anomalies occur—subtle deviations from the expected— which we cannot explain within our traditional scientific framework.[3]

These strange occurrences—as yet scientifically unexplainable, but apparent and recordable—have been called "paranormal." A discipline has arisen to study these human "strangenesses," a facet of psychology called at first "parapsychology" and then "psychoenergetics." It is a mark of the earnestness, the scientific rigor, and the standards of re- search this group set for itself that over ten years ago, in December 1969, the American Association for the Advancement of Science, one of the most respected scientific bodies in the United States, formally included parapsychology as a distinct discipline.

The recognition and understanding of paranormal reality should be part of any truly holistic health practice. It is one of many dimen- sions crucial to our understanding of our patients and our relationship to them. I have on file several dozen descriptions by nurse colleagues of paranormal perceptions which proved accurate: precognitions re- garding their patients' states of health; perceptions that something was physically or emotionally unhealthy about another person despite little or no objective evidence to support the supposition; an uncanny sense that a certain procedure, medication, or therapy was contra- indicated though the patient appeared "as usual." Many of us have had similar experiences, suddenly deciding for no obvious reason to look in on a child, a relative, or a patient to find upon arrival at the bedside that emergency measures were indeed needed.

Precognition can be a useful tool in the assessment of a client's condition, only if the reliability factor is for that particular client truly rather than only statistically, significant. Reliability can be investigated by paying attention to such occurrences in ourselves. With utter regard for the safety of the patient, one can record and practice precognition in even the most traditional health facility. For instance, a record of practice can be gained in assessing patient's condition precognitively by committing one's impressions in writing before having recourse to the patient's laboratory reports or case history, and then later testing these impressions against the hard information. If this is done in a fairly objective manner, there is much to be learned about the subtle cues our interior communication systems send us which we frequently ignore. We can then begin to differentiate, for instance, between a mere guess and an intuition; between a strong "feeling" and an immediate, undeniable, and compulsive conviction. Allowing oneself to explore these types of cues may, in their practiced and mature form, result in a recognition that some of them are reliable sources of congition.

Psychokinesis, the ability to influence matter at a distance, may also play a part in some healing interactions. One place to find it displayed is in the work of mothers or gifted teachers, therapists, or nurses who work with children with cerebral palsy. It is a frequent observation that in the early states of habilitation these children do better at controlling their spastic movements in the presence of certain persons than they do by themselves or in the presence of others. Could it be possible that the former persons, in some as yet undetermined way, influence the "living matter" of these children?

Other factors of the paranormal may influence patient care in ways we do not yet understand. For instance, the hospital experiences of Caribbean people who have come in large numbers to this country in the last decade have been comformed with our expectations about the course of disease that hospitalized them. A significant number of these people appeared only mildly ill on admission but were subsequently beset by a host of confusing and ambiguous symptoms; many of them unexpectedly died. On the other hand, patients seemingly terminal, again without obvious medical "cause," have suddenly become well enough to leave the hospital and return to their normal activities. The frequency of such incidents has aroused considerable interest in the degree to which shamanism and "root" medicine may have influenced the outcome of these patients' cases.

RESEARCH ON HEALING TOUCH

During the past ten years I have engaged in research to develop a valid and reliable therapeutic access to the paranormal through what I have termed "the metaphysics of nursing." I have been particularly interested in healing by "therapeutic touch," a term I coined in 1974 for a method of healing derived from (but not the same as) the laying–on of hands. It is a mode which though present in many cultures has, due to the largely subjective nature of its effect, won little credibility in our modern technological society, where scientific methodologies are based on visible, empirical evidence.

A number of years ago my interest was stimulated when I had the opportunity to participate in some experimental work that was being conducted with a well known healer, Oskar Estebany.[4] My job

was to take the vital signs and record the other psysiological indices
and case histories of the experimental subjects whom Estebany treated
by the laying–on of hands. This gave me an excellent opportunity to
watch the healer closely while he worked on the patients.

What I saw, however, was not remarkable. I saw a man, Estebany,
sit quietly next to a patient and literally lay his hands upon that person
for a varying length of time–usually about 15 to 20 minutes. The atmosphere was quiet and relaxed, and occasionally Estebany would
make small talk to help the patient feel at ease. After 20 minutes or
so, the patient would then leave, and the next day, if warranted, he
or she would return.

There was little to indicate that anything unusual was in progress.
However, when we later followed up these subjects—most of whom
had been medically referred—a greater–than–chance number of the
patients were found to have been considerably improved; some were
apparently cured. These were what could be called bottom–of–the–
barrel patients—people who had been throught the traditional medical
routines without finding succor for their illnesses, most of which were
of a chronic, deteriorating kind. I could not explain these results by
anything in either my previous education or my professional experience. Intrigued by the data, I decided to do an in–depth study of
therapeutic touch.

As in any study, my first recourse was to the literature on touch.
Touch is a primitive sensation. Touch and pain nerve tracts are the
earliest to myelinize in the human fetus central nervous system. In
utero and in its descent through the birth canal, the fetus is exposed
to many cutaneous stimulations. Predictable developmental stages following birth derive their certainty from an evolution of touch experiences: from initial groping hand–mouth explorations which begin
to tell the neonate of the outside world to the development of complex
hand–eye coordination by which it learns to control that environment.
Neonates depend on touch for their initial information. Throughout
life the tips of our fingers and the palms of our hands continue to be
a primary means of sense and perception.

I learned that the touch in which I was interested was not simple
physiological touch, but rather a humanized touch which conveyed
an intent to help or to heal. It needed to be, indeed, suffused with
this motivation. Moreover, the touch was that of fairly healthy persons
whose ego structures were oriented toward serving the patient's needs,
rather than bolstering their own. Such a person would need to understand the phenomenon occurring and act knowledgeably.

As I reviewed the literature, surprisingly little of substantive value had been documented. The most definitive work on therapeutic touch had been done within a biochemical framework. The fundamental studies were completed in the early 1960s by Grad,[5] of McGill University on plants and animals. In these early studies he used the services of Estebany and did several variants of Grad's original research design.

In one series of these studies Grad used a double–blind design to study the effect a healer's hands might have on sprouting barley seeds. He soaked barley seeds first in a saline solution to simulate a "sick" condition in them, and then divided the seeds into three samples. The water with which they were to be irrigated was then treated in the following manner: in the first group the water was taken from the tap; this sample was considered a control group. A second control group was irrigated with water that had come from flasks held by disinterested persons. The third sample was irrigated with water which came from flasks that had been held by Estebany in a manner that simulated what he did when engaged in the laying–on of hands. After five days, it was found that the barley seeds treated by Estebany sprouted earlier, the sprouts grew taller, and they contained more chlorophyll.

In the mid–sixties, a nun–biochemist, Sister M. Justa Smith, became intrigued by Grad's studies. As an enzymologist, she assumed that if an energy change occurred in wound–healing it should be apparent at the enzymatic level, for enzymes are essential to the basic metabolism of living organisms. Estebany again cooperated as the healer, and Sister Justa conducted a double–blind study on the enzyme trypsin. After subjecting the trypsin solution to a high dose of ultraviolet rays to break the chemical bonds, she divided the fresh solution equally into three groups of test tubes: a control group, another group in which the test tubes were subjected to strong magnetic–field radiations, and a group in which the test tubes were held by Estebany in the manner in which he did the laying–on of hands. Repeated trials verified that the chemical activity of the sample held by Estebany were similar to the end of the first hour of treatment. Thereafter, the precisely measured chemical activity of the sample held by Estebany dramatically exceeded those of both the controls and the strong magnetic–field sample.

Sister Justa[6] continued her studies using other enzymes and other healers. She found that all the healers had similar effects on the same enzymes, but that the kind of effect was different on different enzymes. The activity of some enzymes increased, while the activity of others lessened. Still other enzymes seemed to be unaffected. This variability was directly correlated with the individual functions of these enzymes in the body. The change in activity was consistently in the direction of improving or maintaining health.

I found no explanation in the Western scientific literature for this generalized healing effect, so I next studied the philosophy and science of the Orient. The East does indeed claim an understanding of the personalized interaction involved in therapeutic touch. This literature postulates an energy system for which we in the West have neither the word nor the concept. In Sanskrit, it is called "prana," the nearest English translation of which is "vigor" or "vitality." It is that which underlies the organization I call "the life process." According to classical Indian literature[7] there is an overabundance of prana in the healthy individual, whereas the ill person has a deficiency. Indeed, the illness is the deficiency. Prana can be activated by a projection of the will and transferred to another, if the intent to do so is strong. Prana derives from the sun, and the literature appears to indicate that is intrinsic to what in science is known as the oxygen molecule.[7]

As I began to translate this information into a framework consistent with our scientific methodologies, it occurred to me that changes in hemoglobin content might best reflect the effectiveness of the healing process. Hemoglobin, a component of the red blood cells, is necessary for the delivery of oxygen to tissues, and for the processes of electron transport that accompany healing. In Grad's research on the barley seeds, one of the consistent findings in the group treated by Estebany was an increase in chlorophyll content. I knew chlorophyll and hemoglobin were biochemical homologues (tetrapyroles), one of which (chlorophyll) is built around a magnesium atom, the other (hemoglobin) around an iron atom. Since hemoglobin in human metabolism has as central a function as chlorophyll does in plants, I wondered if an increase in health could be correlated with an increase in hemoglobin content. I hypothesized that the healer was an individual whose health gave him access to an abundance of "prana" and whose strong sense of commitment gave him a certain control over the projection of this vital energy for the well being of another. The act of healing, therefore, would entail the channeling of this energy flow by the healer to supplement the deficient energy level of the patient. On a physical level, I suspected that this might occur by electron transfer resonance and that alterations in this resonance would be reflected in the level of the patient's hemoglobin.

Experimental Results

A consideration of the human dynamics involved in studying this phenomenon led me to institute several controls. I controlled for obvious variables such as age (since there is a difference between the hemoglobin values of the very young and the very old); sex (because of the menses, there is a difference in the hemoglobin values of males and females); and drugs, vitamins, and nutritional intakes. I also controlled for persons with histories of unusual changes in blood pressure, temperature, pulse, and respiration in the previous year, and for those who did vigorous exercise or smoked (smoking has an effect on the carboxy–hemoglobin). I also checked certain biorhythms, such as sleep and menstrual cycle, and analyzed the secondary diagnoses of the patients for significant clues for intervening variables. Finally, in the lab tests, I used the hematocrit as a check on the hemoglobin values.

I then did a pilot study based on the hypothesis that there would be significant changes in the hemoglobin values of patients treated by therapeutic touch, whereas there would be no change in the hemoglobin values of patients not so treated. In this study, as in later 1972 and 1973 studies, Estebany was the healer. I used a classical research design with experimental groups (those who were treated by therapeutic touch) and control groups. I hypothesized that there would be a change in the mean hemoglobin value of the experimental group but no significant change in the mean hemoglobin value of the control group. Before the study began, all subjects had their hemoglobin read to assure that comparable groups were being studied and to provide base–line values. Treatment was then instituted, and hemoglobin values were read. This was done again at the end of the course of treatment in the case of the experimental group and after a comparable period in the case of the controls. A confidence level of .01 supported a decision to continue with a full–scale study. This was carried out on an experimental group of 43 subjects and a control group of 33.[8] The findings confirmed the results of the pilot study done in 1971 (p.<.01), and I presented my findings to my colleagues, the American Nurses Association Council of Nurse Researchers, and also to research groups of other professions.

It happened, however, that 1973 was the year Wallace and Benson published their findings on physiological changes in subjects who did transcendental meditation. Although hemoglobin was not one of the variables studied by them, a few persons who critiqued my study felt that the hemoglobin changes I found might be the result of persons in my sample who, unbeknownst to me, followed meditative practices. In addition, it was felt that the hemoglobin changes might be accounted for by respiratory exercise done by some patients following thoracic surgery, or by subjects who engaged in respiratory exercises, such as the pranayamas in yoga.

For these reasons, I replicated the entire study,[9] this time controlling for both meditation and breathing exercises. In this study there were 46 subjects in the experimental group and 29 in the control. The hypotheses were again confirmed, this time at a significance level greater than one in a thousand (p.<.001).

TEACHING THE TECHNIQUE

In the meantime, I had myself been taught the technique of laying–on of hands by Kunz[10] and found, in time, that I achieved with patients results that were similar to those described in the literature. Specifically, when I placed my hands on these patients, they would feel relaxed and after treatment remain so; their hemoglobin values also changed.

I began to suspect that therapeutic touch was a natural human potential which could be done by any person who had a fairly healthy body (creating an overabundance of "prana"), a strong intent to help or heal sick persons, and the ability to learn to project healing intentions to others.

Soon I was instructing registered nurses in the use of therapeutic touch. I tried to help them first to achieve a meditative state in which they could "listen" with their hands as they scanned the bodies of their patients. I then taught them to place their hands on the areas where they sensed or "felt" in the patient's body, to try to redirect energies that seemed to gather there, and to transmit their own feeling of physical well–being to their patients.

In 1974 I designed a research study to see if these nurses could produce the hemoglobin changes that seem to characterize therapeutic touch. This study was done under my direction in hospitals and health facilities in metropolitan New York.[11] In its final form the study included 32 registered nurses and 64 patients in an experimental/control, before/after research design. The experimental group used therapeutic touch. The control group refrained from using it with their patients, that is, they did only routine nursing care.

Because of the nature of this study, I included the following conditions. I requested that each of the participating nurses, whether in the experimental or the control group, abide by the Patient's Bill of Rights—that is, that they have the informed consent of the patient and that they have the cooperation as well as the consent of the patient's attending medical doctor and the department of nursing of the health facility. Where there was a board of research review, I asked that a formal request for approval to use the facilities stipulated that the lab technicians at the health facility not be told that a study was in progress. Consequently those data were derived using the same type of blood–analysis equipment.[12]

The hypothesis were essentially similar to those of the previous studies: that the hemoglobin values of patients in the experimental group would change following treatment by therapeutic touch, whereas the hemoglobin values of comparable patients in the control group would demonstrate no significant difference after a similar period of time. This proved to be the case at a .001 level of significance.

IMPLICATIONS AND PRACTICES

The studies I have quoted by Grad, Sr. Justa, and myself seem to indicate the physiological efficacy of therapeutic touch and to suggest potential for its use. While encouraging others to test these findings and the hypotheses which we have developed to explain them, I began to look into the practical applications of this modality and to inquire whether professionals might be interested in learning about therapeutic touch.[13]

The interest that nurses and other clinicians have expressed in this work has been quite remarkable. In addition to those who regularly participate in the course offered in the Masters Program at the New York University School of Nursing, some 5,000 professional practitioners have attended my workshops in therapeutic touch. Other hospitals and professional schools have expressed interest in finding out what this "new" form of healing is all about. Students trained in therapeutic touch have already begun to introduce it into the curricula in other schools of nursing, two Ph.D. dissertations on therapeutic touch have been completed and accepted as of the date of this writing. Another eight are currently underway.

At present, former students are using therapeutic touch in emergency rooms, in intensive and coronary care units, and in the operating room. Psychiatrists and nurses who work with children and families are teaching family members to perform therapeutic touch on one another, and terminally ill patients are receiving relief from their pain through this modality.

At this time, I do not presume to know either the limitations of therapeutic touch or the dynamics by which it works. I regard my ignorance as an imperative forcing me to try clearly to understand this very ancient and most primitive therapeutic use of the hands. It is only as we learn to integrate our powerful, nonrational capacity for understanding and alleviating illness and restoring balance to the body that we will begin to appreciate not only therapeutic touch but our true potential as human beings. It is a challenge that no person who is committed to healing should fail to appreciate.

REFERENCES

1. Northrup, F. S. C. *The logic of the sciences and the humanities.* New York: Macmillan, 1947.
2. Margenau, H. *The nature of physical reality.* New York: McGraw-Hill, 1950.
3. Kuhn, T. *The structure of scientific revolutions.* Chicago: University of Chicago Press, 1970.
4. Rorvik, D. M. The healing hand of Mr. E. *Esquire,* 1974, *81* (70), 154.
5. Grad, B. A telekinetic effect on plant growth, part 2. *International Journal of Parapsychology,* 1964, *61,* 473–498.
6. Smith, Sister M. Justa. Paranormal Effects on Enzyme Activity. *Human Dimensions,* Spring 1972, *1,* 15–19.
7. Hume, R. E. *The thirteen principal upanishads.* London: Oxford Press, 1921, p. 368.
8. Krieger, D. The response of in–vivo human hemoglobin to an active healing therapy by direct laying–on of hands. *Human Dimensions,* Autumn 1972, *1,* 12–15.
9. Krieger, D. The relationship of touch with intent to help or to heal, to subjects. In–vivo hemoglobin values: a study in personalized interaction. *Proceedings of the American Nurses Association 9th Nursing Research–Conference,* 1973, 39–58.
10. Karagulla, S. *Breakthrough to creativity.* Los Angeles: DeVorss and Co., 1967, pp. 123–146.
11. Krieger, D. Healing by the laying–on of hands as a facilitator of bio-energetic change: The response of in–vivo hemoglobin. *International Journal of Psychoenergetic Systems,* 1976, *1,* 121–129.
12. Krieger, D. Therapeutic touch: The imprimatur of nursing. *American Journal of Nursing,* 1975, *75,* 784–787.

Chapter 9

ACUPUNCTURE: CURRENT STATUS AND CLINICAL RELEVANCE FOR AMERICAN MEDICINE

Michael P. Volen, M.D.
David E. Bresler, Ph.D.

What is the relevance of acupuncture for American medical practice? At present, the views of the medical community toward acupuncture range from enthusiasm[1-4] to complete skepticism.[5-10] It is probably fair to say that most American physicians remain confused about what acupuncture is, and about its clinical applications.

At the UCLA Pain Control Unit, several thousand patients have been treated over the last four years by a number of highly experienced, traditional acupuncturists, chiefly for pain–related problems. On the basis of the results obtained, we have come to accept acupuncture as a valid and effective form of treatment for many medical conditions that have been resistant to current Western medical treatment. This paper will consider the nature of acupuncture, its clinical applications, and its current status in America, and will conclude with our recommendations concerning its appropriate role in American medicine.

History and Traditional Theory of Acupuncture

Sporadic reports of the practice of acupuncture in China have reached the Western world for many years.[11-14] However, not until the last several years has extensive information about acupuncture become available. While it is known that acupuncture originated in China more than three thousand years ago, its origins have been lost in antiquity. As a medical system, its endurance has been remarkable, considering the many cultural and political changes that have swept China. It is quite possible that more people have been treated by acupuncture in the course of human history than by any other formalized system of medicine.

The ancient Chinese believed that the universe is permeated with a vital life energy ("ch'i") thought to circulate constantly through all living organisms. This energy was thought to follow specific pathways through the body, referred to as "meridians," upon which the various acupuncture "points" lie. There are twelve bilaterally symmetrical meridians, each of which is named for a major internal organ, plus two control meridians that traverse the midline of the body, one dorsally and one ventrally. Altogether there are several hundred acupuncture points on the body.

According to traditional Chinese thought, pain or disease are somatic manifestations of an imbalance caused by the blockage of energy flow through the body. This imbalance can result from either external physical causes or internal psychological factors. By careful examination of the patient, the traditional acupuncturist attempts to diagnose the nature of the imbalance of energy, and then correct it through stimulation of appropriate acupuncture points. The selection of specific points and the type of technique used are determined by rather complex theoretical considerations. Years of study are required for the traditional acupuncturist to master the theoretical basis of the art, as well as to learn the precise location of each acupuncture point and numerous needle–manipulation techniques.

At its most sophisticated level, acupuncture is considered a form of preventive medicine, which may be utilized for the maintenance of health, as well as for the treatment of disease. It is said that accomplished traditional acupuncturists can detect disturbances in the homeostasis of the organism even before they are manifested as overt disease. Thus this ancient form of Chinese medicine approaches patients in a way that emphasizes the state of the whole person, rather than just the alleviation of symptoms.

MODERN CONCPTS OF ACUPUNCTURE

Although the terminology of traditional Chinese medicine often appears strange and unfamiliar to Western physicians, scientists have now begun to document the physiological, electrical, and chemical characteristics inherent in the traditional acupuncture system. Many acupuncture points are anatomically identical to motor points of muscles, well–known in electromyography, while others are identical to common trigger points, independently described by several Western investigators.[15–17] Still others lie along major nerve trunks.[18,19] Most interestingly, it has been found that the electrical resistance of the skin overlying acupuncture points is considerably lower than that of the surrounding area,[20–22] although the significance of this observation has yet to be explained. While basic research on acupuncture in the West has not been extensive, it has been shown that stimulation of various acupuncture points can affect a great variety of physiological parameters. These include changes in red and white blood cell count, immunoglobulin levels, EEG and EKG recordings, bronchodilatation, and vasodilatation of the microcirculation among others.[23–35]

Most theories of acupuncture have focused on the nervous system, and it seems clear that the phenomena of acupuncture are at least in part mediated by the nervous system, through mechanisms not as yet well understood. Neurophysiological investigations of acupuncture have concentrated upon its analgesic effects, which various theories developed have attempted to explain. The existence of visceral–cutaneous reflexes and characteristic patterns of referred pain are well–known, and it is possible that acupuncture may involve in part a complex manipulation of such reflexes.[36–43] Melzack and Wall have advanced the well–known "gate theory"[44] and others have amplified this with "multiple gate" theories.[45–46] Basically, these theories propose that needle insertion at acupuncture points stimulates large–diameter fibers in peripheral nerves, the activity of which interferes at some level of the nervous system with the transmission of painful impulses mediated by small–diameter fibers. The impulses produced by acupuncture thus close the "gate" to impulses mediating painful stimuli and prevent them from reaching the brain.

No single explanation of the phenomena has been generally accepted, and it is quite possible that a number of different factors may be involved, including peripheral neural stimulation, immune–inflammatory response to the needle insertion, and psychological factors.[47] Quite recently, the discovery of endogenous polypeptides (endorphins) which bind to opiate receptors[48-50] in the central nervous system has raised the intriguing possibility that release of these polypeptides may also be involved in mediating the analgesic effect of acupuncture.[51,52]

Endorphins are naturally occurring substances with opiatelike properties, whose analgesic actions can be reversed by opiate antagonists, such as naloxone. Preliminary investigations indicate that the analgesic effects of acupuncture may also be blocked by naloxone,[53,54] which suggests the existence of a similar mechanism.

ACUPUNCTURE TREATMENT

How is acupuncture actually performed? Basically a typical treatment involves the insertion of several solid, fine gauge, flexible stainless steel needles. The needles are inserted to a depth ranging from a few millimeters to three to six centimeters, depending upon the particular point chosen and the physique of the individual patient. The number of needles inserted at each treatment may range from two or three to 20 or 30 or even more, depending upon the problem under treatment, and the style of the individual acupuncturist. An average treatment involves the use of approximately eight to twelve needles.

Following insertion, the needles may simply be left in place, or they may be manipulated in a variety of ways. For stronger stimulation, they may be gently twirled by hand, or they may be connected to an "electroacupuncture" device which delivers a low, painless electrical current through the needles. They may also be heated by burning the Chinese herb "moxa" (the dried leaves of Artemisia vulgaris), traditionally used for this purpose.

Although any procedure involving needle insertion into the body holds a potential for danger, we have found that acupuncture is extremely safe in the hands of well–trained therapists, who observe appropriate precautions and contraindications. At the UCLA Pain Control Unit, over 30,000 acupuncture treatments have been administered by both physicians and traditional acupuncturists without a single major complication.

CLINICAL APPLICATIONS OF ACUPUNCTURE

At present, the most common application of acupuncture is for treatment of chronic pain problems. Despite numerous medical and surgical techniques available, management of chronic pain is often unsatisfactory, as is reflected in the countless prescriptions written for analgesics, muscle relaxants, tranquilizers, and anti–inflammatory agents. Acupuncture represents a different approach to pain relief for many patients, with none of the potential problems associated with surgery or long–term drug therapy.

Approximately 4,000 patients, most of them with chronic pain problems, have been treated at UCLA over the last six years. Patients with many different medical conditions have been treated, and many have experienced significant and long–lasting relief from pain. A detailed discussion of these results is beyond the scope of this paper, but we will indicate some general findings.

Slightly more than one–half of a study group of 400 patients with a wide range of pain problems experienced significant pain relief, with decreased requirements for medications, improved sleep patterns, and increased ability to carry on daily activities. This study group was composed of patients who had run the gamut of conventional treatment and whose pain problems were unresponsive to standard therapy.

Some types of pain problems appear to respond better than others to acupuncture. It is effective in relieving many types of musculoskeletal pains, such as arthritis, bursitis, tenosynovitis, vertebrogenic pain, and other similar conditions. Patients with osteoarthritis generally respond much more favorably than those with rheumatoid arthritis. Perhaps this is related to the fact that rheumatoid arthritis is actually a multisystem disease while osteoarthritis is a local degenerative process. There also appear to be anatomical differences in the pattern of response, and problems of the large joints commonly respond better than those of the smaller joints. For example, the pain of bursitis or tenosynovitis of the shoulder is often relieved successfully and rapidly by acupuncture, while epicondylitis of the elbow responds more slowly.

Acupuncture appears to be particularly effective when there is a large component of muscle spasm involved. It can produce rapid and dramatic relief of spasm and can be quite useful in the treatment of acute musculoskeletal injuries. The application of acupuncture to sports medicine may prove to be especially successful.

Headaches, both tension and migraine, can also be effectively treated by acupuncture. It can produce relief of acute headache pain, and can eventually eliminate or markedly diminish the recurrence of headaches after completion of a full course of treatment.

The pain of various neurological conditions may also respond well to acupuncture. Included are such disorders as peripheral neuropathy, trigeminal neuralgia, postherpetic neuralgia, phantom limb pain, and causalgia, extremely painful conditions for which no satisfactory form of treatment now exists. While such treatments are not always successful, many patients have been helped substantially, and acupuncture should therefore be considered as a possible form of treatment for these conditions. Indeed, for disorders such as true trigeminal neuralgia—an agonizing condition unresponsive to most therapy—acupuncture may well be the treatment of choice, as in many cases it attenuates the intensity and frequency, and in some cases entirely eliminates, the pain.

One final pain problem that deserves specific mention is temporomandibular joint (TMJ) dysfunction. This is a problem usually treated by dentists, although it may be seen by some physicians. Not well understood by many members of both professions, its management is somewhat controversial and often unsatisfactory. Acupuncture has been found to be particularly effective in the treatment of this problem, especially when used in conjunction with soft diet and other appropriate adjunctive measures. TMJ dysfunction has a surprisingly high incidence, but often goes unrecognized or is misdiagnosed. Acupuncture represents a very promising form of therapy for this problem.

Many other kinds of pain problems may also respond well to acupuncture treatment and we will not enumerate them further. It must be remembered, of course, that acupuncture should be used for pain relief only when a clear diagnosis has been established. Pain is often a symptom of an underlying disease which requires treatment and it may be possible to mask pain by the inappropriate use of acupuncture. Thus one would no more administer acupuncture to a patient with undiagnosed acute abdominal pain than one would an injection of morphine. The same principles of sound medical judgment apply to the use of acupuncture as to any other means of producing analgesia.

We believe that acupuncture for the treatment of chronic pain should no longer be considered an "experimental" technique, for when administered by well–trained therapists, it can be a highly effective means of pain control. Nevertheless, there is nothing magical about acupuncture, and it is not a cure–all for every patient. Some patients treated with acupuncture obtain little or no relief.

Chronic pain is a complex phenomena; it is a sensation, a perception, and an emotion, the experience of which is determined by the interaction of many physical and psychological factors.[55] Many patients with chronic pain develop extensive secondary gains from their problem, which make them unwilling on some level to become cured of their pain. Chronic pain or illness may be a means of obtaining affection or attention, of avoiding responsibility, of financial gain, or of many other forms of satisfaction. In these cases, acupuncture must be combined with appropriate psychological management in order to be maximally effective.

OTHER INDICATIONS FOR ACUPUNCTURE

What other clinical applications are there for acupuncture? Acupuncture is employed by traditional physicians in China for everything from the common cold to acute appendicitis to schizophrenia. However, it has not been administered to significant numbers of patients in this country for anything other than pain control. We now enter a more speculative area, though in descriptions of the more promising areas for acupuncture treatment that follow, much of the information remains anecdotal.

Some patients with asthma and/or allergic rhinitis appear to respond well to acupunture. Most people with uncomfortable plugged nostrils due to allergic rhinitis experience prompt and dramatic clearing of their breathing immediately following treatment. However, it is not clear whether there is real long–term improvement or only temporary symptomatic relief. Some asthmatic patients have also shown clinical improvement with acupuncture treatment, and controlled studies performed at UCLA have shown that acupuncture can partially reverse acute methacholine–induced bronchospasm.[34] Perhaps there will be a role for acupuncture in the management of chronic asthmatics, allowing them to decrease their dependence upon drugs and minimize the adverse effects often associated with long–term drug therapy. This possibility needs further investigation.

Various neurological disorders have been treated with acupuncture, including tremors, both secondary to Parkinsonism and of unknown etiology, involuntary tics and torticollis, spasticity related to demyelinating disorders such as multiple sclerosis, and various sequelae of brain and spinal cord damage, such as problems of bladder and bowel control, and impotence. This is a disparate group of disorders about which it is difficult to generalize, but they indicate the type of problem for which acupuncture may be tried. They are, for the most part, conditions for which no satisfactory treatment is now available. They are also difficult to treat with acupuncture and therefore the results have been inconsistent. However, some patients have responded well, and in view of the lack of alternatives, a trial of acupuncture may be indicated for certain patients with these kinds of problems.

The treatment of nerve deafness by acupuncture in China has generated considerable interest, but results in this country have not been encouraging.[56] Although some patients and their families have reported subjective improvement, there have been no objective changes observed by audiometric examination following treatment. The explanation for this is not clear and it is conceivable that acupuncture may affect some aspect of hearing not well measured by audiometric testing. However, at present, acupuncture cannot be considered an effective treatment for nerve deafness.

The traditional Chinese concept of balancing opposing energies in the body appears analogous to the idea of balancing the sympathetic and parasympathetic divisions of the autonomic nervous system. For example, many "functional" gastrointestinal ailments can be thought of in terms of autonomic imbalance and they often respond favorably to acupuncture. Various cardiovascular, gastro–intestinal, metabolic, and other illnesses may be represented in terms of autonomic dysfunction; these disorders may also be amenable to acupuncture therapy.

The foregoing applications of acupuncture have received minimal attention in America, and there is thus a need for much broader clinical investigation of acupuncture in areas other than the treatment of chronic pain.

ACUPUNCTURE IN THE TREATMENT OF PSYCHOLOGICAL DISORDERS

A significant number of Americans suffer from some manifestation of anxiety/depression, and there is reason to believe that acupuncture may be a helpful form of therapy. It is an interesting observation that most patients receiving acupuncture report feelings of relaxation and well–being, and even occasional mild euphoria following their treatment. This nonspecific effect of acupuncture seems to be unrelated to the particular problem being treated, and may perhaps involve release of endogenous opiates.

Certain kinds of treatment and certain acupuncture points appear to be more powerful in inducing this relaxation response. It is unclear why this relaxation occurs, but anyone who regularly employs acupuncture recognizes it as a typical response to therapy. Many patients who begin treatment dreading the needles eventually come to regard their acupuncture treatment as a curiously pleasant experience, and occasionally patients will be disappointed when they are told that it is time to end their treatments. In addition to changes in specific symptoms, it is also fairly common for patients to report feeling less anxious and more energetic, and sleeping better. Undoubtedly, this plays a part in the improvement of many chronic pain patients, most of whom suffer anxiety and depression as a consequence of their chronic illness.

Various compulsive disorders may be treated by acupuncture, and it has been employed in the treatment of obesity, withdrawal from drugs, and cigarette smoking. Very tiny needles are inserted at acupuncture points in the ear, sometimes remaining in place for several days. It must be made clear that acupuncture in no way causes the obese patient to lose weight. Instead, it appears to minimize the feelings of hunger which occur when a restricted diet is successfully followed. Appetite remains the same and strong psychological motivation is required for success. Similarly, acupuncture will not make someone want to stop smoking, but will decrease the physical discomfort resulting from abstention from cigarettes.

Many patients will testify that acupuncture has helped them, and it is difficult to say whether it produces a physiological effect or functions as an effective form of suggestion. Quite possibly both are involved. Because of the great interest among the general public in new ways of losing weight or stopping smoking, this area holds great possibilities for unscrupulous practitioners. Thus the limitations of these techniques should be carefully explained, and it should be made clear that acupuncture in no way constitutes an easy or magical way for the unmotivated individual to lose weight or stop smoking.

ACUPUNCTURE PRACTICE IN AMERICA

Acupuncture is extensively utilized in China, often in conjunction with Western medicine, for a wide variety of medical, surgical, and psychological problems. It is also widely practiced in Japan, Korea, and throughout much of the Orient, as well as in the Soviet Union and Eastern and Western Europe, where it is generally recognized as an accepted form of treatment. However, acupuncture has still not become generally utilized in America. According to the American Medical Association, acupuncture is not yet a proven therapeutic modality and its use at this time must therefore be considered "experimental." In view of this position, Medicare, Medicaid, and many insurance carriers will not pay for acupuncture treatment. Thus to a large extent, acupuncture is now available only to those who can afford to pay for it or who have insurance policies that include coverage for acupuncture.

The legal and political status of acupuncture also remains confused, with widely differing laws regulating the practice of acupuncture being passed by different state legislatures. Many states permit the practice of acupuncture only by licensed physicians, but those who wish to include acupuncture in their practice are often faced with dramatically increased malpractice insurance rates.

The patient who wishes to receive acupuncture in America is often faced with a difficult situation. Many individuals claim to be acupuncturists, but in the absence of a system of regulation and licensure, the prospective patient has no reliable means of choosing a competent practitioner. Often the recommendations of friends or neighbors who have received successful treatment may be the best guide available.

Many patients prefer to consult a physician for acupuncture, but a medical degree is no guarantee of expertise in acupuncture. In the last few years there has been a proliferation of acupuncture courses for physicians and other health care professionals, which consist of a few days or a weekend of training. These may provide a worthwhile introduction to the subject, but are not sufficient training for participants to begin the clinical practice of acupuncture. More extensive teaching programs are needed for physicians who wish to incorporate acupuncture into their medical practice.

ACUPUNCTURE RESEARCH IN AMERICA

To create a more favorable situation for the practice of acupuncture, further clinical investigations of its efficacy will be necessary. Studies at UCLA and elsewhere have obtained positive results in the use of acupuncture, but some other investigators have reached negative conclusions. In interpreting these results, it is important to understand the difficulties inherent in acupuncture research.

In order for any form of therapy to be effective, it must be administered properly. For example, if we wished to evaluate the effectiveness of penicillin for the treatment of streptococcal infections, and gave our subjects a single penicillin tablet with breakfast for four days, we would undoubtedly conclude that it was worthless, or at best, minimally effective. In order to work, penicillin must be used in the proper dosage according to the proper schedule, and for a sufficient period of time. The same is true with acupuncture. The proper points must be used, they must be stimulated correctly, and a sufficient number of treatments must be administered if we expect to observe positive results.

Many studies of acupuncture performed in this country have been done by individuals with no formal training in acupuncture, who simply followed instructions from a textbook. Not surprisingly, results in this kind of situation have been disappointing. For example, when acupuncture is administered correctly, the patient experiences a mild paresthesia or characteristic tingling, aching sensation. The experienced acupuncturist eventually develops a feeling for the proper placement of the needles to routinely evoke this sensation. A less experienced therapist may need to rely upon careful probing with the needle until the patient responds with this sensation.

However, some studies performed by Western physicians without training in acupuncture have consisted of the placement of acupuncture needles at the approximate location and depth of points described in acupuncture texts. No attempt is made to elicit the sensation of paresthesia, which is the only assurance of proper needle placement. The acupuncture points must be located precisely and slight variations exist from one individual to the next. Needle insertion which only approximates their location cannot be expected to have a significant effect, and studies of this kind do not provide a valid appraisal of acupuncture.

Other studies by Western physicians inexperienced in acupuncture therapy have provided insufficient treatment either in the number of points stimulated, or the number of treatments administered. This may be due to the experimenters' unfamiliarity with patterns of patient response to acupuncture, which may vary considerably. Some patients experience a gradual improvement in symptoms following each treatment, while others notice no change for several treatments before improvement starts to occur. Still others experience a transient exacerbation of symptoms after some initial treatments preceding eventual improvement. Long–term worsening of symptoms as a result of acupuncture does not seem to occur.

Because of this variability, it is quite difficult to generalize as to the number of treatments that may be required for a given individual. As a very rough estimate, we consider ten treatments a fair trial of acupuncture for most pain problems. In general, patients who will respond to acupuncture should begin to show a response within this time, although there may be exceptions in particularly stubborn cases. Of course, some individuals may require considerably more than ten treatments for maximum improvement, while others may experience complete relief before they have even reached ten treatments. Some patients also find an occasional "booster" treatment helpful nine to twelve months following a full course of treatment.

In the light of this pattern of response, one must question the significance of studies in which only a small number of treatments are provided. For example, a study of acupuncture consisting of four treatments at which three needles are inserted may show no improvement in the subjects. If these same patients were treated by an experienced acupuncturist, they might require eight or ten treatments with stimulation of a dozen acupuncture points before showing a significant response.

An additional variable in acupuncture research is the type of stimulation employed. An experienced acupuncturist will decide on an individual basis whether mild or vigorous stimulation is appropriate, and whether manual stimulation of needles, massage, burning of moxa (moxibustion), or electrical current will produce the best results. As are other forms of medicine, acupuncture is an art, and its effectiveness cannot be adequately judged by investigators unfamiliar with its intricacy who simply insert needles in the skin on the basis of a standardized protocol.

Thus the many American investigators attempting to evaluate acupuncture without sufficient knowledge of the subject to perform their studies properly yield poor results inducing portions of the medical community to adopt a negative, skeptical attitude toward acupuncture. While it is certainly important to protect the public against medical quackery, can we really believe that a medical system employed for thousands of years by one–quarter of the world's population and now growing in acceptance throughout the world is really quackery? At any given time in history, people tend to cling to accepted beliefs and resist the introduction of new ideas. We look back with amusement at the narrowmindedness of past generations, but must take care that we ourselves do not react in the same way. Acupuncture represents an exciting opportunity for American physicians, and should not be rejected because it is unfamiliar and appears strange compared to accepted medical practice. Although we do not fully understand acupuncture, we make use of other techniques and drugs, such as aspirin or digitalis, whose mechanism of action is also not completely understood.

Surprisingly, patients do not seem to find the idea of acupuncture as strange as do many physicians. It is actually more comprehensible to them than many of the modern procedures of Western medicine, and patient acceptance of acupuncture is usually quite good. They are willing to try acupuncture if it will help them, and physicians may approach it in the same way, as a means of treating patients whom they were previously unable to help.

CONCLUSION

We believe that the best interest of Americans is served by allowing experienced nonphysician acupuncturists to practice legally. Most Oriental traditional acupuncturists in this country are not licensed health professionals, yet they possess the greatest skill in acupuncture. If acupuncture is to be made available to the general public, certainly those most expert in the field should be permitted to perform it. This is not to say that any person claiming to be an acupuncturist should be licensed to practice. All persons applying to be licensed as acupuncturists should be required to furnish proof of thorough training and experience, and be required to pass an examination in the theory and practice of acupuncture, as well as demonstrate sufficient knowledge of anatomy and physiology and familiarity with aseptic techniques.

In examining the long–range future of acupuncture, it would be appropriate to consider it a part of the practice of medicine, and as such, the province of physicians and other licensed health professionals. However, if physicians are to perform acupuncture, they must be adequately trained in its use. At the present time, few such opportunities for legitimate training exist. In the future, we would hope to see acupuncture being taught as a part of the curriculum of medical and dental schools, as well as on a postdoctoral level for physicians wishing to develop additional clinical skills. We would also hope to see serious continuing education programs in the field of acupuncture offered to physicians already in practice.

Will any of this occur while acupuncture is considered an "experimental" procedure by organized medicine? It seems unlikely that it will, yet many investigators in the field of acupuncture now believe that there is more than sufficient evidence to consider acupuncture beyond the level of "experimental." Certainly this is so for treatment of chronic pain problems. Further clinical investigation of acupuncture is necessary, and research findings should be carefully evaluated by the medical profession so that the judgment of "experimental" may be removed from the practice of acupuncture in many clinical situations.

The introduction of acupuncture to America represents an important and exciting opportunity for physicians and other health–care professionals. We hope that the medical profession will not turn its back upon acupuncture, but will approach it with a positive attitude and a willingness to consider new ideas and concepts. On the basis of our experience at UCLA, we believe that there are many millions of Americans suffering from conditions that could be helped by acupuncture treatment. Now is the time for health–care professionals to begin making this safe and effective form of therapy available to them.

REFERENCES

1. Dimond, E.G. Acupuncture anesthesia—Western medicine and Chinese traditional medicine. *Journal of the American Medical Association,* 1971, *218,* 1558–1563.
2. Sidel, V. The barefoot doctors of the People's Republic of China. *New England Journal of Medicine,* 1972, *286,* 1292–1300.
3. Sidel, V. Medical education in the People's Republic of China. *The New Physician,* 1972, *21,* 284–293.
4. Tkach, W. I have seen acupuncture work. *Today's Health,* 1972, *50,* 50–56.
5. Kroger, W.S. Hypnotism and acupuncture. *Jounral of the American Medical Association,* 1972, *220,* 1012–1013.
6. Kroger, W.S. Acupuncture analgesia: Its explanation by conditioning theory, autogenic training and hypnosis. *American Journal of Psychiatry,* 1973, *130,* 855–860.
7. Wall, P. Acupuncture revisited. *New Scientist,* October 3, 1974, pp. 31–34.
8. Taub, A. Acupuncture in the treatment of intractable pain. *The Lancet,* September 15, 1973, p. 618.
9. DeBakey, M.D. A critical look at acupuncture. *Reader's Digest,* September 1973, pp. 137–140.
10. Chaves, J. F., & Barber, T.X. Hypnotic procedures and surgery: A critical analysis with applications to "Acupuncture Analgesia." *American Journal of Clinical Hypnosis,* 1976, *18,* 217–236.
11. Acupuncturation. *The Lancet,* November 1823, pp. 200–201.
12. Banks, J.T. Observations on acupuncture. *Edinborough Medical and Surgical Journal,* 1831, *35,* 323.
13. Churchill, J.M. *A treatise on acupuncture.* London: Simpkin and Marshall, 1821.
14. Stevens, T.J. Sciatica treatment by acupuncture. *Boston Medical and Surgical Journal,* 1869, *2,* 392.

15. Liu, Y.K. The correspondence between some motor points and acupuncture loci. *American Journal of Chinese Medicine*, 1975, *3*, 347–358.
16. Melzack, R., Stillwell, D.M., & Fox, E.J. Trigger points and acupuncture points for pain: Correlations and implications. *Pain*, 1977, *3*, 3–23.
17. Vanderschot, L. Trigger points vs. acupuncture points. *American Journal of Acupuncture*, 1976, *4*, 233–238.
18. Shanghai Medical College Acupuncture Anesthesia Group. Study of relations between the acupuncture points and surrounding nervous structure by anatomical dissection. *Liberation Daily News*, January 5, 1972.
19. Matsumoto, T., & Lyu, B.S. Anatomical comparison between acupuncture and nerve block. *The American Surgeon*, January 1975, pp. 11–16.
20. Reichmanis, M., Marino, A.A., & Becker, R.O. Electrical correlates of acupuncture points. *IEEE Transactions on Biomedical Engineering*, November 1975, pp. 533–535.
21. Becker, R.O., Reichmanis, M., Marino, A.A., & Spadaro, J.A. Electrophysiological correlates of acupuncture points and meridians. *Psychoenergetic Systems*, 1976, *1*, 105–112.
22. Reichmanis, M., Marino, A.A. & Becker, R.O. D.C. skin conductance variation at acupuncture loci. *American Journal of Chinese Medicine*, 1976, *4*, 69–72.
23. Chen, K.C. Effects of electroacupuncture on the immunological reactions of rabbits to goat plasma anticoagulant factor. Sansi Acupuncture Symposium (Report #103) Sansi China, April 1959.
24. Chen, K.C. Effects of Acupuncture & Electroacupuncture on Immunological Reactions. Sansi Acupuncture Symposium (Report #102). Sansi, China, April 1959.
25. Yang, K.C. et al. Relationship between acupuncture—moxibustion & infection and immunity. In Yu, H. & Hsieh, S.W. (Eds.), *Advances in immunity.* Shanghai: Shanghai Science & Technology Press, 1962, p.140.
26. Craciun, T., Toma, C., & Turdeanu, V. Neurohumoral modification after acupuncture. *American Journal of Acupuncture*, 1973, *1*, 67–70.
27. Omura, Y. Effects of acupuncture on blood pressure, leukocytes & serum lipids & lipoproteins in essential hypertension. *Federation Proceedings*, 1974, *33*, 430.
28. Lung, C.H., Sun, A.C., Tsao, C.J., Chang, Y.L., & Fan, L. An observation of the humoral factor in acupuncture analgesia in rats. *American Journal of Chinese Medicine*, 1974, *2*, 203–205.
29. Chu, Y.M., & Affronti, L.F. Preliminary observations on the effect of acupuncture on immune responses in sensitized rabbits & guinea pigs. *American Journal of Chinese Medicine*, 1975, *3*, 151–163.
30. Hu, J.H. Therapeutic effects of acupuncture: A review. *American Journal of Acupuncture*, 1974, *2*, 8–14.

31. Bresler, D.E Electrophysiological and behavioral correlates of acupuncture therapy. In Z. Reidak (Ed.); *Konference o Vyzkumu Psychotroniky*. Prague: Sbornik Referatu, 1973.

32. Wen, H.L. & Chan, K. Status asthmaticus treated by acupuncture and electrostimulation. *Asian Journal of Medicine*, 1973, *9*, 191–195.

33. Calehr, H. Acupuncture treatment of the asthmatic patient. *American Journal of Acupuncture*, 1973, *1*, 41–51.

34. Tashkin, D.P., Bresler, D.E., Kroening, R.J., Kerschner, H., Katz, R.L., & Coulson, A. Comparison of real and simulated acupuncture and isoproterenol in methacholine–induced asthma. *Annals of Allergy*, 1977, *39*, 379–387.

35. Lee, G.T.C. A study of electrical stimulation of acupuncture locus tsusanli (ST–36) on mesenteric microcirculation. *The American Journal of Chinese Medicine*, 1974, *2*, 1–27.

36. Tien, H.C. Acupuncture anesthesia: Neurogenic interference theory. *World Journal of Psychosynthesis*, 1972, *4*, 36–41.

37. Tien, H.C. Neurogenic interference theory of acupuncture anesthesia. *American Journal of Chinese Medicine*, 1973, *1*, 105.

38. Ionescu–Tirgoviste, C. Theory of mechanism of action in acupuncture. *American Jounral of Acupuncture*, 1973, *1*, 193–199.

39. Looney, G.L. Acupuncture study. *Journal of the American Medical Association*, 1974, *228*, 1522.

40. Chang, H.T. Integrative action of the thalamus in the process of acupuncture for analgesia. *American Journal of Chinese Medicine*, 1974, *2*, 1–39.

41. Mann, F. *Acupuncture—The ancient Chinese art of healing and how it works scientifically*. New York: Random House, 1974.

42. Wancera, I., & Konig, G. On the neurophysiological explanation of acupuncture analgesia. *American Journal of Chinese Medicine*, 1974, *2*, 193–198.

43. Small, T.J. The neurophysiological basis for acupuncture. *American Journal of Acupuncture*, 1974, *2*, 77–87.

44. Melzack, R., & Wall, P. Pain mechanisms: A new theory. *Science*, 1965, *150*, 971.

45. Man, P.L., & Chen, C.H. Mechanisms of acupuncture anesthesia: Two gate theory. *Disease of the Nervous System*, 1972, *33*, 730.

46. Melzack, R. How acupuncture can block pain. *Impact of Science on Society*, 1973, *23*, 65–75.

47. Bresler, D.E., & Kroening, R.J. Three essential factors in effective acupuncture therapy. *American Journal of Chinese Medicine*, 1976, *4*, 81–86.

48. Hughes, J., Smith, T.W., Kosterlitz, H.W., Fothergill, L.A., Morgan, B.A., & Morris, H.R. Identification of two related pentapeptides from the brain with potent opiate agonist activity. *Nature* (London), 1975, *258*, 577–579.

49. Terenius, L., & Wahlstrom, A. Search for an endogenous ligand for the opiate receptor. *Acta Physiologica Scandinavia*, 1975, *94*, 74–81.

50. Cox, B.M., Ophiem, K.E., Techmacher, H., & Goldstein, A. A peptide-like substance from the pituitary that acts like morphine. *Life Sciences*, 1975, *16*, 1777–1785.

51. Pomeranz, B. Brain opiates at work in acupuncture? *New Scientist*, January 6, 1977, pp. 12–13.

52. Sjohund, B., Terenius, L., & Eriksson, M. Increased cerebrospinal fluid levels of endorphins after electroacupuncture. *Acta Physiologica Scandinavia*, 1977, *100*, 382–384.

53. Pomeranz, B.H., & Chiu, D. Naloxone blocks acupuncture analgesia and causes hyperanalgesia: Endorphin is implicated. *Life Sciences*, 1976, *19*, 1757–1762.

54. Mayer, D.J., Price, D.D., & Rafii, A. Antagonism of acupuncture analgesia in man by the narcotic antagonist naloxone. *Brain Research*, 1977, *121*, 368–372.

55. Bresler, D.E. *Free yourself from pain.* New York: Simon & Schuster, 1979.

56. Eisenberg, L., Taub, H.A., & DiCarlo, L. Acupuncture therapy of sensorineural deafness. *New York State Journal of Medicine*, October 1974, pp. 1942–1949.

Part IV

INTEGRAL
MEDICINE IN ILLNESS

C. Norman Shealy is a neurosurgeon, O. Carl Simonton a radiation oncologist. During the early 1970s, each became disillusioned with the therapeutic modalities—surgery, drugs, and radiation—that their specialties offered. Both began to explore ways in which the mind would cause or cure physical illness, and each began to develop ways to mobilize his patients' own capacity to relieve pain or to combat cancer. By the middle of the decade, Dr. Shealy had created a Pain and Rehabilitation Center in La Crosse, Wisconsin, and Dr. Simonton and his wife, Stephanie Matthews, had opened the Cancer Counseling and Rehabilitation Center, a nonprofit organization dedicated to the study and treatment of the emotional aspects of cancer, located in Fort Worth, Texas.

Dr. Shealy is currently director of the Pain and Health Rehabilitation Center in Springfield, Missouri and founding president of the American Holistic Medical Association. Dr. Shealy has lectured and published extensively on the subject of chronic pain and is the author of *The Pain Game* (Celestial Arts, 1976), *90 Days to Self Health* (Dial Press), and *To Parent or Not* (Downing, 1980).

Chapters 10 and 12 in this section outline some of the factors which caused Drs. Shealy and Simonton to abandon their profession's conventional wisdom, describe some of the techniques they have used to mobilize their patient's psychophysiological responses, and detail some aspects of the programs they have created to treat chronic pain and widely disseminated cancer. The Simontons' essay, which is reprinted by permission, has also appeared in their book, *Getting Well Again.*

O. Carl Simonton, M.D., is medical director of the Cancer Counseling and Research Center, former chief of Radiation Therapy, Travis Air Force Base, noted lecturer and teacher, and is associated with the Bresler Center Medical Group in West Los Angeles, California.

Dr. Simonton developed a unique approach to cancer treatment, combining meditation, guided imagery, and biofeedback techniques with more traditional medical approaches. For the past seven years he has researched and evaluated the effects of various psychological modalities that can influence the course of malignancy.

Stephanie Matthews–Simonton is program director at the Cancer Counseling and Research Center. She is responsible for the development and implementation of the intensive counseling program used to study those highly selected patients who have significantly outlived their life expectancy. She has also worked as cotherapist with Dr. Simonton in facilitating group therapy sessions with cancer patients.

Chapter 10

A COMPREHENSIVE HEALTH–ORIENTED PAIN–CONTROL PROGRAM

C. Norman Shealy, M.D., Ph.D.

By 1963, when I completed a residency in neurosurgery, I was already convinced that its procedures were not effective for managing benign, intractable pain. Over the next several years, research into the neurophysiology of the central nervous system helped guide me to my present approach to pain control. Investigations in the early 1960s found that painful stimuli induced prolonged firing throughout the entire spinal cord, except in the posterior columns. In 1965 Melzack and Wall published their theory on the gate control of pain.[1] Briefly, the Melzack–Wall theory stated that there is normally a balance between large sensory fibers (beta fibers) and the smaller sensory fibers (C fibers). When the C fibers are excessively activated or the beta fibers are destroyed, pain spontaneously occurs. Acute pain might occur from the tensing of nerve fibers, pressure upon them, or burning them. Chronic pain, on the other hand, is more likely to be due to a disturbance in the ratio between the two fiber systems. Thus C fibers that lack the modulation of the beta fibers spontaneously cause pain.

The only area in the entire nervous system where beta fibers and C fibers are separated is in the dorsal columns. Stimulation of the dorsal columns might lead to pain relief.[2] In the spring of 1967, two

137

years after I began my theoretical work, I first implanted a dorsal–column stimulator in a patient.[3] Over the next four years I implanted stimulators in some 40 patients selected from a large number of people with various kinds of chronic pain.

From the time I began my work, however, it was obvious to me that many patients had serious personality flaws that interfered with their ability to respond to a mechanical device for relieving pain. Minnesota Multiphasic Personality Inventories (MMPI's), the surgeon's clinical opinion, and psychiatric evaluations were obtained on patients who were considered candidates for the procedure. These three screening procedures revealed that 94 percent of the patients with chronic pain had psychological profiles which would prevent them from obtaining much benefit from dorsal–column stimulation. Since only 6 percent of the chronic–pain patients were candidates for dorsal–column stimulation, and since no known treatment was available for the other 94 percent, I began in 1971 to look for other ways to manage relief for chronic–pain patients.

In 1971 I visited Wilbert Fordyce's behavioral modification program at the University of Washington. I saw that when Fordyce treated one or two patients in an intense behavior modification program for two months he was able to withdraw 60 percent of them from drugs while affording them marked symptomatic relief. Unfortunately, only about one–third of the total number of patients maintained this improvement at follow–up six months after discharge. Still, this safe, noninvasive, behavioral approach seemed to constitute a remarkable improvement over traditional medicine and surgery.

PAIN–CONTROL TREATMENT PROGRAM

In the fall of 1971, borrowing from Fordyce's treatment and from a variety of other approaches, I opened in LaCrosse, Wisconsin, what I believe was the first comprehensive pain–control treatment program. The initial program consisted of the following:

Behavior modification: Carried out in the hospital in a special 25–bed unit, behavior modification involved nursing personnel, who simply ignored pain complaints, behavior that indicated pain, and "painful body language."

Drug withdrawal: Carried out in a systematic fashion, withdrawal took place in the following way: patients' narcotics were converted to Methadone; aspirin and Tylenol were substituted for Darvon and similar drugs; and sodium amytal replaced various tranquilizers. All of these were then withdrawn systematically in a routine fashion. It was found that all patients could be withdrawn within two weeks, without serious withdrawal symptoms, and that only 10 percent of the patients missed the drugs when they were withdrawn.

Progressive physical exercise: Normal limbering of joints, muscles, and tendons was carried out in a progressive way; guided exercises were required twice each day. Prescribed distances for walking and times for stationary bike–riding were also recommended.

Massage: Total body massage was carried out two or three times each week by a masseur. In addition, the nurses and aides on the floor carried out vigorous slapping massage of the area of pain, followed by an ice rubdown four times a day. A mechanical vibrator was also used once or twice a day.

Heat: Hydrocollator packs were used over painful areas prior to the total body massage, and whirlpool baths were used twice a day on each patient.

Ice: Ice rubdowns, as well as Therapac(R)* (a self–applied ice pack which melts within 20 minutes) were found to be even more effective than heat.

Transcutaneous electrical nerve stimulation (TENS):   Used from the beginning of the program, initially, only with the available ancient device dating from 1918. More recently, modern external electrical stimulators have been adapted by the program.

Acupuncture: Available and quite helpful for 10 percent of patients with chronic, benign pain, acupuncture was somewhat helpful for another 15 percent. However, we learned that 90 percent of the patients who responded well to acupuncture responded equally well or better to TENS.

Swimnastics: Calisthenic exercises in the swimming pool five days a week added a great deal of fun to the physical–limbering program. Unfortunately, most patients have limited access to continuing this activity at home.

---

*There is no direct or implied endorsement for any product or proprietary intended in this article. Products mentioned were used as the only available choice at the mentioned time.

Nutrition: Attention to diet has always been part of the program. We have emphasized that patients should avoid sugar, caffeine, and nicotine and should eat a well–balanced diet with a wide variety of foods and a fresh salad every day.

Dorsal–Column Stimulation: During the first year, we continued to recommend implantation of a stimulator to the 6 percent of patients whom we felt might benefit most from it. Gradually, however, as the successes of other parts of the program mounted, we restricted the use of stimulators. We have not recommended this in over five years.

Psychotherapy: For the first year, each patient was seen by a psychiatrist in group therapy three mornings a week. These group–therapy sessions, however, seemed to subvert our behavior–modification program. They allowed too much negativity and hostility to be manifested and were therefore discontinued.

Facet rhizotomy: In the spring of 1972, a procedure was devised for denervating painful joints in the back. Facet rhizotomy was done initially with radio–frequency current, and later with an injection of a 4 percent solution of phenol in glycerine. This procedure has become an accessory to the total program.

At the end of the first year, our major improvement on the Fordyce behavior–modification program was a decrease in average patient stay to one month rather than two months. In addition, 80 percent of our patients were markedly better at the end of the one–month period, a 33 percent improvement over simple behavior–modification.

Patients are told that drugs are considered detrimental to their ability to gain control over their pain. We suggest that they ask us to write a drug–withdrawal schedule for them, but patients are not forced into drug withdrawal unless they wish it. Reading the patients the complications of each of their drugs from the *Physician's Desk Reference* has proven most useful in convincing them to reduce or eliminate drug consumption.

The various mechanical therapies that are feasible in an out patient situation are continued. TENS, acupuncture, ice, massage, heat, and physical exercise are all important parts of the treatment program.

Biofeedback

All patients are given biofeedback training, primarily with temperature biofeedback. It is emphasized to them that their capacity for learning to control the circulation in the fingertips is only an indication of the degree to which they can control all body functions. Examples such as childhood training in bladder and bowel control are used. They are taught also that patients with 7th nerve palsies who have been treated with 11th or 12th nerve transplants, standing in front of a mirror training themselves to have a normal voluntary smile, are themselves using a kind of biofeedback to expedite their learning. These examples, plus demonstrations to the patients that they can learn to raise their temperature within a day or two, are effective in giving them faith in their own ability to control body function.

Biogenics (R)

A very elaborate mental–exercise program has been devised synthesizing components from progressive relaxation, autogenic training,[5] autosuggestion,[7] Jungian symbolic exercises, and psychosynthesis.[8]

The system that has been devised emphasizes that a positive attitude is necessary but not sufficient for pain control, that deep muscular relaxation is essential for mental regulation of the body but is not by itself adequate. Physiologic balancing of body functions is also necessary; patients who are relaxed may not always have a balanced autonomic nervous system nor be free from psychosomatic "blocks"— areas of the body which cannot be felt or which feel numb. Patients are, accordingly, taught to feel each part of their body and its sensations independently and then to balance each part of the body with all other parts.

To supplement this physiologic balancing, psychological balancing is taught, a process whereby each patient consciously and intelligently comes to grips with the serious conflicts within his or her life which in some cases may have contributed to, or be perpetuating, the illness. For instance, a woman with a five–year history of rheumatoid arthritis, reported that her arthritis was no longer present after seven days of the various psychological insight–balancing exercises. On the 12th day, she gave the following story: "I'm 50 years old, and I've been married 28 years. During all this time, my husband has been unfaithful to me. When our children were younger, I promised myself that when our third child was 18 and had left home, I would divorce my husband. When our third son was 18, however, he was drafted and sent to Viet Nam with his two brothers. I could not divorce their father while they were in Viet Nam. When my sons came home safely from Viet Nam, I could not divorce their father because I was an invalid and he was taking care of me. And I kept saying to myself, if it were not for that son–of–a–gun, I would not have this disease. But a few days ago, I

suddenly realized that it was not my husband's fault that I had rheumatoid arthritis; it was my anger towards him that was destroying my
body." She made a conscious, intelligent decision to forgive her husband for his infidelity. She decided she would not get divorced since
he treated her well and loved her and since she just didn't feel like
starting over again. Four years after this insight—and the emotional
balancing which followed it—she is still free of rheumatoid arthritis
both clinically and by laboratory tests.

Once the patient has adequately developed the conviction that he
or she can be well, has learned to relax, and has learned physiologic
and psychologic balancing, then "special programming" is used. Special
programming consists of a personal healing phrase or "physiologic
mantra," such as "My back is flexible and comfortable," accompanied
by a visualization in which the desired goal is attained. Patients practice
these techniques while in the clinic for about eight hours a day—four
to five hours while guided by a staff member, and three to four hours
on their own with tapes. During the rest of the clinic day patients
receive the various mechanical therapies and intensive personal counseling.

The final stage of the Biogenics program is spiritual attunement.
Schultz[5] noted that after about six months of autogenic training many
patients begin spontaneously to meditate, a process which he felt led
to attunement with God or the Divine. Many of the exercises we use
in the pain–control program are designed to help the patients seek
spiritual attunement, to help put them in touch with their own inner
self or ideal goals.

THE CENTER

About 200 patients can be seen in a given year at the Pain and
Health Rehabilitation Center. This allows us to work with new patients
every three weeks, while permitting the staff one week to see old patients, catch up on administrative and paper work, etc. Actually, we
prefer to see patients two weeks out of every four with two weeks for
study, research, and catching up.

The patients range in age from 20 to 84 years, most patients being
between 35 and 50. Sixty percent of them are female and about 35
percent have had Workmen's Compensation injuries. Most patients
are of middle–class background. Indeed, the most difficult patients
we have had to treat have been the few millionaires who have been
through the program. Doctor's wives have also presented unusual
challenges.

Sixty percent of the patients have had previous lumbar surgery, an average of four to five operations per patient. Ten percent of patients have had chronic back pain, sometimes with sciatica, but have never had operations on their backs. Approximately 10 percent have either migraine or tension headaches. The remaining 20 percent present every conceivable form of chronic pain, usually pain from some previous injury or surgical procedure, but sometimes spontaneous pain, such as tic douloureux, atypical facial neuralgia, postherpetic pain—all of which seem to respond to the program.

All patients are evaluated at admission and upon discharge according to their "pain profile" (Table 1). Their total score is added so that a maximum abnormal score is 500 and a perfect score 0. At the end of the two–week session, 90 percent of all patients show a 50 to 100 percent reduction in their pain profile scores. Patients who follow the Biogenics and physical–exercise program outlined for them

Table 1
Pain Profile

On the columns below, grade yourself (circle) on these factors:
  a. Your average severity of pain (100 = intolerable, excruciating, horrible);
  b. Effect of pain upon physical activity. How much is your physical activity reduced or cut down by pain. (0 = none, 100 = totally incapacitated);
  c. The average percent of time pain is felt;
  d. Effect of your illness on your mood or personality (100 = totally withdrawn, panicked, overwhelmingly depressed);
  e. Drugs consumed (M.D. will complete this item based on scores for each drug prescribed)

a	b	c	d	e
Average Pain	Average Physical Activity	Percentage of Time Pain is Felt	Effect on Mood	Average Drug Consumption
0	0	0	0	0
5	5	5	5	5
10	10	10	10	10
15	15	15	15	15
20	20	20	20	20
25	25	25	25	25
30	30	30	30	30
35	35	35	35	35
40	40	40	40	40
45	45	45	45	45
50	50	50	50	50
55	55	55	55	55
60	60	60	60	60
65	65	65	65	65
70	70	70	70	70
75	75	75	75	75
80	80	80	80	80
85	85	85	85	85
90	90	90	90	90
95	95	95	95	95
100	100	100	100	100

when they go home tend to be most likely to continue to improve during the year following discharge.

Initially, in the hospital–based program, only 60 percent of the patients were doing well after one year. However, in our most recent follow–up, 72 percent of the patients maintained their improvement or continued to get better during the year after they left the program. In fact, 84 percent of all patients who practiced Biogenics are improved 50 to 100 percent. A few patients have improved lastingly from the use of TENS, acupuncture, or facet rhizotomy during the two weeks with us. Of those patients improved at six months, 98 percent remain improved two years later at two–year follow–ups.

During the last four years, we are increasingly seeing patients with problems other than pain: cancer, asthma, high blood pressure, etc. These people seem to respond to our program just as well as chronic–pain patients. It appears that chronic disease, in general, often represents a disturbance in both the physiology and the psychology of the individual, that any successful therapy must address itself to all aspects of patient's lives—physical, mental, emotional, and spiritual—to help them achieve the balance that is health.

CONCLUSION

Over the past ten years, our treatment program for chronic–pain patients has evolved from surgical implantation of electrical stimulating devices to an intense, holistically oriented program in which patients are treated physically, emotionally, mentally, and spiritually. A variety of mechanical techniques are used, but the most important part of the therapeutic work is self–regulatory training in which the intention is to bring physical and emotional functions into balance under the patient's voluntary control. The desired state of mind consists of a positive attitude, a belief that healing can occur, relaxation, physiologic balancing, psychological balancing, special reprogramming, and spiritual attunement. It is suggested that, if this kind of training were given to people in general, health maintenance would be enhanced.

REFERENCES

1. Melzack, R. & Wall, P.D. Pain mechanisms: A new theory. *Science,* 1965, *150,* 971–979.
2. Shealy, C.N., Taslitz, N., Mortimer, J.T., & Becker, D.P. Electrical inhibition of pain: Experimental evaluation. *Anesthesia and Analgesia. Current Researches,* 1967, *46,* 299–305.

3. Shealy, C.N., Mortimer, J.T., & Reswick, J.B. Electrical inhibition of pain by dorsal column stimulation: Preliminary clinical report. *Anesthesia and Analgesia. Current Researches*, 1967, *46*, 489–491.

4. Fordyce, W.E., Fowler, R.S., Lehmann, J.F., & Delateur, B.J. Some implications of learning in problems of chronic pain. *Journal of Chronic Disability*, 1968, *21*, (179), 90.

5. Schultz, J.H., & Luthe, W. *Autogenic therapy*. Volumes I–IV. New York: Grune and Stratton, 1969.

6. Shealy, C.N. *Health: A workbook of biogenic exercises*. Pain and Health Rehabilitation Center, La Crosse, 1975.

7. Coue, E. *How to practice suggestion and autosuggestion*. New York: American Library Service, 1976.

8. Assagioli, R. *Psychosynthesis*. New York: Viking Press.

Chapter 11

A PSYCHOPHYSIOLOGICAL MODEL FOR INTERVENTION IN THE TREATMENT OF CANCER

O. Carl Simonton, M.D.
Stephanie Matthews–Simonton

Why do some patients recover their health and others die, when the diagnosis is the same for both? Carl became interested in this problem while he was completing his residency as a cancer specialist at the University of Oregon Medical School. There he noticed that patients who stated they wanted to live would often act as if they did not. There were lung cancer patients who refused to stop smoking, liver cancer patients who wouldn't cut down on alcohol, and others who wouldn't show up for treatment regularly.

In many cases, these were people whose medical prognosis indicated that, with treatment, they could look forward to many more years of life. Yet while they affirmed again and again that they had countless reasons to live, these patients showed a greater apathy, depression, and attitude of giving up than did a number of others diagnosed with terminal disease.

This paper is excerpted from the book *Getting Well Again*, by O. Carl Simonton, M.D., Stephanie Matthews–Simonton and James Creighton. (J.P. Tarcher, Inc., 1978).

146

In the latter category was a small group of patients who had been sent home after minimal treatment, with little expectation that they would live to see their first follow–up treatment. Yet several years later, they were still arriving for their annual or semiannual examinations, remaining in quite good health, and inexplicably beating the statistics.

When Carl asked them to account for their good health they would frequently give such answers as, "I can't die until my son graduates from college," or "They need me too much at work," or "I won't die until I've solved the problem with my daughter." The common thread running through these replies was the belief that they *exerted some influence over the course of their disease.* The essential difference between these patients and those who would not cooperate was in their attitude toward their disease and their positive stance toward life. The patients who continued to do well, for one reason or another, had a stronger "will to live." This discovery fascinated us.

Stephanie, whose background was in motivational counseling, had an interest in unusual achievers—those people in business who seemed destined to go to the top. She had studied the behavior of exceptional performers and had taught the principles of that behavior to average achievers. It seemed reasonable to study cancer patients in the same way—to learn what those who were doing well had in common, and how they differed from those who were doing poorly.

If the difference between the patient who regains his health and the one who does not is, in part, a matter of attitude toward the disease and belief that he could somehow influence it, then, we wondered, how could we influence patients' beliefs in that positive direction? Might we be able to apply techniques from motivational psychology to induce and enhance a "will to live"? Beginning in 1969, we began looking at all the possibilities, exploring such diverse psychological techniques as encounter groups, group therapy, meditation, mental imagery, positive thinking, motivational techniques, "mind development" courses such as Silva Mind Control and Mind Dynamics, and biofeedback.

From our study of biofeedback, we learned that certain techniques were enabling people to influence their own internal body processes, such as heart rate and blood pressure. An important aspect of biofeedback, called visual imagery, was also a principal component of other techniques we had studied. The more we learned about the process, the more intrigued we became.

Essentially, the visual–imagery process involved a period of relaxation during which the patient would mentally picture a desired goal or result. With the cancer patient, this would mean his attempting to visualize the cancer, the treatment destroying it and, most importantly, his body's natural defenses helping him recover. After discussions with two leading biofeedback researchers, Drs. Joe Kamiya and Elmer Green, of the Menninger Clinic, we decided to use visual–imagery techniques with cancer patients.

The first patient with whom an attempt was made to apply our developing theories was a 61–year–old man who came to the medical school in 1971 with a form of throat cancer that carried a grave prognosis. He was very weak, his weight had dropped from 130 pounds to 98 pounds, he could barely swallow his own saliva, and was having difficulty breathing. There was less than a 5 percent chance that he would survive five years. Indeed, the medical school doctors had seriously debated whether to treat him at all, since it was distinctly possible that therapy would only make him more miserable without significantly diminishing his cancer.

Carl went into the examining room determined to help this man actively participate in his treatment. This was a case that justified using exceptional measures. Carl began treating the patient by explaining how the patient himself could influence the course of his own disease. Carl then outlined a program of relaxation and mental imagery based on the research we had been accumulating. The man was to set aside three, five– to fifteen–minute periods during the day—in the morning on arising, at noon after lunch, and at night before going to bed. During these periods he was first to compose himself by sitting quietly and concentrating on the muscles of his body, starting with his head and going all the way to his feet, telling each muscle group to relax. Then, in this more relaxed state, he was to picture himself in a pleasant, quiet place—sitting under a tree, by a creek, or anywhere that suited his fancy, so long as it was pleasurable. Following this he was to imagine his cancer vividly in whatever form it seemed to take.

Next, Carl asked him to picture his treatment, radiation therapy, as consisting of millions of tiny bullets of energy that would hit all the cells, both normal and cancerous, in their path. Because the cancer cells were weaker and more confused than the normal cells, they would not be able to repair the damage, Carl suggested, and so the normal cells would remain healthy while the cancer cells would die.

Carl then asked the patient to form a mental picture of the last and most important step—his body's white blood cells coming in, swarming over the cancer cells, picking up and carrying off the dead and dying ones, flushing them out of his body through his liver and kidneys. In his mind's eye he was to visualize his cancer decreasing in size and his health returning to normal. After he completed each such exercise, he was to go about whatever he had to do the rest of the day.

What happened was beyond any of Carl's previous experience in treating cancer patients with purely physical intervention. The radiation therapy worked exceptionally well, and the man showed almost no negative reaction to the radiation on his skin or in the mucous membranes of his mouth and throat. Halfway through treatment he was able to eat again. He gained strength and weight. The cancer progressively disappeared.

During the course of treatment—both radiation therapy and mental imagery—the patient reported missing only one mental–imagery session on a day when he went for a drive with a friend and was caught in a traffic jam. He was most upset, both with himself and with his friend, for in missing just that one session he felt his control over his condition was slipping away.

Treating a patient in this way was very exciting, but it was also somewhat frightening. The possibilities for methods of healing that seemed to be opening up before us went beyond anything that Carl's formal education had prepared him for.

The patient continued to progress until finally, two months later, he showed no signs of cancer. The strength of his conviction that he could influence the course of his own illness was evident when, close to the end of his treatment, he said to Carl, "Doctor, in the beginning I needed you in order to get well. Now I think you could disappear and I could still make it on my own."

It is fortunate that the results of this first case were as dramatic as they were, for as we began to talk openly in medical circles about our experiences and to put forward the idea that patients had a much larger influence over the course of their disease than we gave them credit for, we received strong negative reactions. Indeed, there were many times when we, too, doubted our own conclusions. Like everyone else—and particularly anyone with medical training—we had been taught to see illness as "happening" to people, without any possibility of individual psychological control over its course, or little cause–effect relationship between the illness and what was going on in the rest of their lives.

However, we continued to use this new approach to cancer. Although it sometimes made no difference in the illness, in most cases it made significant changes in patients' responses to treatment. Today, in the more than seven years since Carl worked with that first patient, we have evolved a number of other processes in addition to mental imagery that we have used with patients, first at Travis Air Force Base, where Carl was chief of radiation therapy, and now at the Cancer Counseling and Research Center in Fort Worth.

A Whole–Person Approach to Cancer Treatment

Because cancer is such a dread disease, the minute people know someone has cancer, it often becomes the person's defining characteristic. The individual may play numerous other roles—parent, boss, lover—and have numerous valuable personal characteristics—intelligence, charm, a sense of humor—but from that moment on he or she is a "cancer patient." The person's full human identity is lost to his or her cancer identity. All anyone is aware of, often including the physician, is the physical fact of cancer, and all treatment is aimed at the patient as a body, not as a person.

It is our central premise that an illness is not purely a physical problem but rather a problem of the whole person, that it includes not only body but mind and emotions. We believe that emotional and mental states play a significant role both in susceptibility to disease, including cancer, and in recovery from all disease. We believe that cancer is often an indication of problems elsewhere in an individual's life, problems aggravated or compounded by a series of stresses six to eighteen months prior to the onset of cancer. The cancer patient has typically responded to these problems and stresses with a deep sense of helplessness or "giving up." This emotional response, we believe, in turn triggers a set of physiological responses that suppress the body's natural defenses and make it susceptible to producing abnormal cells.

Assuming our beliefs are essentially accurate, it then becomes necessary for patient and physician in working toward recovery to consider not only what is happening on a physical level but, just as importantly, what is going on in the rest of the patient's life. If the total integrated system of mind, body, and emotions, which constitute the whole person, is not working in the direction of health, then purely physical interventions may not succeed. An effective treatment program, then, will deal with the total human being and not focus on the disease alone.

A HISTORICAL LOOK AT THE CONNECTION BETWEEN CANCER AND EMOTIONS

The connection between cancer and emotional states has been observed for nearly 2000 years. In fact, it is the separation of cancer from emotional states that is the new and strange idea. Writing nearly 2000 years ago in the second century A.D., the physician Galen observed that cheerful women were less prone to cancer than were women of a depressed nature.[1] Gendron, in a treatise written in 1701 inquiring into the nature and causes of cancer, cited the influence of the "disasters of life as occasion much trouble and grief."[2]

In 1783 Burrows, in a comment that sounds remarkably like an early description of chronic stress, attributed the disease to "the uneasy passions of the mind with which the patient is strongly affected for a long time."[3]

In 1865 Dr. Claude Bernard wrote a classic text, *Experimental Medicine*,[4] in which he reported observations similar to our own. Bernard cautioned that a living being must be considered as a harmonious whole. Although separate analysis of body parts was necessary for investigation, he said, the relations among the parts must also be considered. And, in another classic text, *Surgical Pathology*,[5] published in 1870, Sir James Paget expressed his conviction that depression plays a vital role in the occurrence of cancer:

> The cases are so frequent in which deep anxiety, deferred hope, and disappointment are quickly followed by the growth and increase of cancer that we can hardly doubt that mental depression is a weighty additive to the other influences favouring the development of the cancerous constitution.

The first statistical study of emotional states and cancer was undertaken in 1893 by Snow. In reporting this relatively sophisticated research in *Cancers and the Cancer-Process*,[6] Snow concluded that:

> Of all causes of the cancer–process in every shape, neurotic agencies are the most powerful. Of the most prevalent kinds, distress of mind is the one most commonly met with; exhausting toil and privation ranking next. These are direct exciting causes that exert a weighty predisposing influence towards the development of the rest. Idiots and lunatics are remarkably exempt from cancer in every shape.

Despite the apparent agreement among late nineteenth– and early twentieth–century experts that there was a connection between emotional states and cancer, interest waned in the face of general anesthesia, newly developing surgical procedures, and radiation therapy. The success of these physical therapies with many medical problems substantially strengthened the viewpoint that physical problems could be solved only with some form of physical treatment. In addition, physicians began to see stresses such as hard work and privation as inevitable; after all, even if they did play a role in the onset of cancer, what could a physician do about them? Finally, until the first third of the twentieth century the tools for dealing with emotional problems were still quite limited.

Yet it is one of the ironies of medical history that, as the emerging sciences of psychology and psychiatry developed the diagnostic tools to test the link between cancer and emotional states scientifically and the therapeutic tools to assist in dealing with emotional problems, medicine lost interest in the problem. The result has been two very distinct bodies of literature and research. The psychological literature is rich with descriptions of the emotional states related to cancer, but it often fails to suggest any physiological mechanisms that might explain this relationship. The medical literature is well–grounded in physiology but, perhaps because it does not integrate psychological data into its research, it is unable to explain "spontaneous" remission or major differences in how individuals respond to treatment.[7]

Coming from a medical background, Carl was startled to find substantial evidence of the links between emotional states and cancer in the psychological literature. We have since observed that few physicians are aware of this research. The price of this age of specialization is that persons in different disciplines working on the same problem often have little exchange of information. Each discipline develops its own specialized language, its own values, and its own method of communicating information; important information can be lost because the disciplines do not exchange findings effectively.

THE PSYCHOLOGICAL EVIDENCE

One of the finest studies on emotional states and cancer was reported in *A Psychological Study of Cancer,*[8] written in 1926 by Dr. Elida Evans, a Jungian psychoanalyst, with an introduction by Carl Jung. Jung wrote that he believed Evans had solved many of the mysteries of cancer—including why the course of the disease is not always predictable, why the disease can sometimes recur after many years with no sign of illness, and why it is a disease associated with industrialized society.

Based on her analysis of 100 cancer patients, Evans concluded that many cancer patients had lost an important emotional relationship before the onset of the disease. She saw such patients as people who had invested their identity in one individual object or role (a person, a job, a home) rather than developing their own individuality. When the object or role was threatened or removed, such patients were thrown back on themselves, with few internal resources for coping. (We, too, have found the characteristic of putting others' needs before one's own in our patients, as you will see in the case histories that follow.) Evans also believed that cancer was a symptom of other unresolved problems in a patient's life, and her observations have since been confirmed and elaborated on by a number of other researchers.

Dr. Lawrence LeShan, an experimental psychologist by training and a clinical psychologist by experience, is the foremost theorist of the psychological life history of cancer patients. In his recently published book, *You Can Fight for Your Life: Emotional Factors in the Causation of Cancer,*[9] he reports findings similar in many ways to those of Evans. LeShan identifies four typical components in the life histories of the more than 500 cancer patients with whom he worked:

1. The patient's youth was marked by feelings of isolation, neglect, and despair, with intense interpersonal relationships appearing difficult and dangerous.

2. In early adulthood, the patient was able to establish a strong, meaningful relationship with a person, or found great satisfaction in his or her vocation. A tremendous amount of energy was poured into this relationship or role. Indeed, it became the reason for living, the center of the patient's life.

3. The relationship or role was then removed—through death, a move, a child leaving home, a retirement, or the like. The result was despair, as though the "bruise" left over from childhood had been painfully struck again.

4. One of the fundamental characteristics of these patients was that the despair was "bottled up." These individuals were unable to let other people know when they felt hurt, angry, hostile. Others frequently viewed the can-

cer patients as unusually wonderful people, saying of
them: "He's such a good, sweet man" or "She's a saint."
LeShan concludes "The benign quality, the 'goodness'
of these people was in fact a sign of their failure to
believe in themselves sufficiently, and of their lack of
hope."

He describes the emotional state of his patients after they lost the
crucial relationship or role as follows:

> The growing despair that each of these people faced appear[s]
> to be strongly connected with the loss that each suffered in child-
> hood . . . . they saw the end of the relationship as a disaster that
> they had always half expected. They had been waiting for it to
> end, waiting for rejection. And when it happened, they said to
> themselves, "Yes, I knew it was too good to be true." . . . From a
> superficial point of view, all managed to "adjust" to the blow. They
> continued to function. They went about their daily business. But
> the "color," the zest, the meaning went out of their lives. They
> no longer seemed attached to life.
>
> To those around them, even people close to them, they
> seemed to be coping perfectly well . . . but in fact it was the false
> peace of despair that they felt. They were simply waiting to die.
> For that seemed the only way out. They were ready for death. In
> one very real sense they had already died. One patient said to
> me, "Last time I hoped, and look what happened. As soon as my
> defenses were down, of course I was left alone again. I'll never
> hope again. It's too much. It's better to stay in a shell."
>
> And there they stayed, waiting without hope for death to re-
> lease them. Within six months to eight years, among my patients,
> the terminal cancer appeared.

LeShan reports that 76 percent of all the cancer patients he interviewed shared this basic emotional life history. Of the cancer patients who entered into intensive psychotherapy with him, over 95
percent showed this pattern. Only 10 percent of a control group of
noncancer patients revealed this pattern.[10]

Although LeShan writes movingly and convincingly of his patients'
emotional states, not all facets of his observations have yet been validated by other studies. But several key elements have been confirmed
by a thirty–year study by Caroline B. Thomas, a psychologist at Johns
Hopkins University.

Dr. Thomas began interviewing medical students at Johns Hopkins in the 1940's and evaluating their psychological profiles. Since

then, she has interviewed more than 1300 students and followed their history of illness. She reports that the most distinctive psychological profile belonged to students who subsequently developed cancer— more distinctive even than that of students who subsequently committed suicide. In particular, her data showed that students who subsequently developed cancer saw themselves as having experienced a lack of closeness with their parents, seldom demonstrating strong emotions, and being generally low gear.[11]

Another element of LeShan's description, that cancer patients tend to be prone to feelings of hopelessness and helplessness even before the onset of their cancer, has been confirmed by two other studies.

> Drs. A.H. Schmale and H. Iker observed in their female cancer patients a particular kind of giving–up, a sense of hopeless frustration surrounding a conflict for which there was no resolution. Often this conflict occurred approximately six months prior to the cancer diagnosis. Schmale and Iker then studied a group of healthy women who were considered to be biologically predisposed to cancer of the cervix.
>
> Using psychological measures that allowed them to identify a "helplessness–prone personality," in this group Schmale and Iker predicted which women would develop cancer—and were accurate 73.6 percent of the time. The researchers pointed out that this does not mean that feelings of helplessness *cause* cancer—these women appeared to have some predisposition to cervical cancer—but that the helplessness seemed to be an important element.[12]
>
> Over a period of 15 years, Dr. W.A. Greene studied the psychological and social experiences of patients who developed leukemia and lymphoma. He too observed that the loss of an important relationship was a significant element in the patient's life history. For both men and women, Greene said, the greatest loss was the death or threat of death of a mother; or for men, a "mother figure," such as a wife. Other significant emotional events for women were menopause or a change of home; and for men, the loss or threat of loss of a job, and retirement or the threat of retirement.[13]

Greene concluded that leukemia or lymphoma developed in an environmental setting in which the patient had dealt with a number of losses and separations that produced a psychological state of despair, hopelessness, and discontinuity.

Other studies have confirmed LeShan's description of the difficulty many cancer patients experience in expressing negative feelings and the need to constantly look good to others.

> Dr. D. M. Kissen has observed that the major difference between heavy smokers who get lung cancer and heavy smokers who do not is that the lung cancer patients have "poorly developed outlets for emotional discharge."[14]
>
> E. M. Blumberg demonstrated that the rate of tumor growth can be predicted based on certain personality traits. The patients with fast–growing tumors attempted to give a good impression of themselves. They were also more defensive and less able to defend themselves against anxiety. In addition, they tended to reject affection, even though they wanted it. The slow–growing tumor group showed a greater ability to absorb emotional shocks and to reduce tension by physical activity. The difficulty for the patients with fast–growing tumors seemed to be that the emotional outlets were blocked by an extreme desire to make a good impression.[15]
>
> Dr. B. Klopfer conducted a similar study in which tumor type (fast or slow growth) was predicted based on personality profiles. The variables that allowed the researchers to predict rapid growth were patients' ego defensiveness and loyalty to "their own version of reality." Klopfer believes that when too much energy is tied up defending the ego and the patient's way of seeing life, the body will not have the necessary vital energy to fight the cancer.[16]

In addition to the studies cited, experience with our patients leaves no reasonable doubt in our minds of a link between certain emotional states and cancer.

These connections between stress, personality and illness have been elaborated over and over in many ways. Our aim has been to use this information to develop means of intervening in the disease process with the intent of assisting a person in their fight toward better health.

RELAXATION AND MENTAL IMAGERY

Relaxation and mental imagery are among the most valuable tools we have found to help patients learn to believe in their ability to recover from cancer. In fact, we mark as the conception of our present approach the first time Carl used mental imagery with a patient. Since then, we have discovered that mental imagery is not only an effective motivational tool for recovering health, but is also an important tool for self–discovery and for making creative change in other areas of life.

We owe our discovery of the relaxation and mental–imagery process to Stephanie's background in motivational psychology. Because of her training, we were aware that this process for altering expectations had been used by people in many different disciplines. The common thread running through these disciplines was that people created mental images of desired events. By forming an image, a person makes a clear mental statement of what he or she wants to happen. And, by repeating the statement, he or she soon comes to expect that the desired event will indeed occur. As a result of this positive expectation, the person begins to act in ways consistent with achieving the desired result and, in reality, helps to bring it about.

For example, a golfer would visualize a beautiful golf swing with the golf ball going to the desired place. A business person would visualize a successful business meeting. A stage performer would visualize a smooth opening night. A person with a malignancy would picture the tumor shrinking and the body regaining health.

As we were learning the effectiveness of the relaxation and mental imagery process, we were also learning of the evidence that biofeedback researchers were amassing that people could learn how to control inner physiological states, such as heart rate, blood pressure, and skin temperature.[17] When interviewed, these people frequently stated that they had not been able to command the body to alter the internal state but instead had learned a visual and symbolic language by which they communicated with the body.

We first began using mental imagery to motivate patients and provide them with a tool for influencing their immune systems, but we soon discovered that the activity revealed extremely important in-

formation about patients' beliefs. This discovery was somewhat acci-
dental. When we first began assigning the mental imagery process,
we would ask our patients whether they were practicing it regularly,
but we did not try to ascertain *what* their imagery was. However, when
one patient's condition went steadily downhill, even though he steadfastly maintained he was using the process three times a day, we asked
him specifically to describe the content of his imagery.

His answer confirmed our fears. When asked what his cancer
looked like, he said, "It looks like a big black rat." When asked how
he envisioned his treatment, which consisted of chemotherapy in the
form of small yellow pills, he replied, "I see the little yellow pills going
into my bloodstream, and once in a while the rat eats one of these
pills." Asked what happened when the rat ate the pills, he said, "Well,
he's sick for a while, but he always gets better, and then he bites me
all the harder." When we asked about his white blood cells imagery,
he replied, "They look like eggs in an incubator. You know how eggs
sit under the warm light? Well, they're incubating in there, and one
day they're going to hatch."

The imagery paralled his deteriorating condition. First of all, the
cancer was strong and powerful—a "big black rat." The treatment was
weak and impotent, "tiny pills" that the rat ate only occasionally and
that had only a temporary effect on him. Finally, the white blood cells,
the representatives of his body's natural defenses, were completely
immobile. Our patient had created an almost perfect image of total
suppression of the immune system and had been faithfully repeating
this imagery three times a day.

We soon discovered that other patients also showed strongly negative expectancies in their imagery. One patient reported that, "I visualize my cancer as a big rock. Every once in a while, these little scrub
brushes come to clean up around the edges of the rock, but they can't
do much good." Again, the cancer appeared strong and impregnable
while the body's defenses were puny and impotent, unable to "do much
good."

Another patient reported that he saw his white blood cells "as a
snowstorm that sweeps over my whole body and obliterates most of
the cancer cells in a single pass, but a few pop back." Here the body's
defenses appeared to be more potent, but they did not really destroy
the cancer cells, they only glossed over them. Moreover, since snow-
flakes have no directionality or intelligence, this imagery revealed that
the patient did not see his body's defenses as actually recognizing and
destroying the cells: Their impact was by sheer numbers.

These experiences made us realize how important it was to examine the contents of our patients' imagery closely to see what expectancies were being communicated. Since then, we have used the significance of the imagery to determine whether patients show a general pattern of glossing over or trying to hide negative feelings, or otherwise impede their treatments.

The imagery process is an important and very powerful part of the program. However, it is only one tool that has been developed to influence the mind and body in support of treatment. The first step in getting well is to understand how beliefs and emotional responses have contributed to illness.

THE PSYCHOLOGICAL PROCESS OF ILLNESS

From our experience and from the research of others, we can identify five steps of a psychological process that frequently precedes the onset of cancer.[18]

1. *Experiences in childhood result in decisions to be a certain kind of person.* Most of us remember a time in childhood when our parents did something we didn't like and we made an internal pledge: "When I grow up I'm never going to be like that." Or a time when some contemporary or adult did something that we regarded highly and we made an internal pledge to behave in a similar way whenever we could. Many of these childhood decisions are positive and have an overall beneficial effect on our lives; many, on the other hand, do not.

Our main concern is with the decisions made in childhood which limit a person's resources for coping with stresses. By adulthood, most of these childhood decisions are no longer conscious. The same ways of acting have been repeated so many times that awareness of our ever having made a choice is lost. But unless these choices are changed, they become the rules of the game of our life. Every need to be met, every problem to be solved must be handled within these limited choices made in early childhood.

Most of us tend to see ourselves as being the way we are just because "that's the way we are." But when the history of our choices is made conscious, new decisions can be made.

2. *The individual is rocked by a cluster of stressful life events.* Both the research and our own observations of patients indicate that major stresses are often a precursor to cancer. Frequently, clusters of stresses occur within a short period of time. The critical stresses we have identified are those that threaten personal identity, perhaps including the

death of a spouse or loved one, retirement, or the loss of a significant role.

3. *These stresses create a problem with which the individual does not know how to deal.* It is not just the stresses that create the problem, but the inability to cope with the stresses given the "rules" about the way he or she has to act and the role decided upon in early life. When the man who is unable to permit himself close relationships, and therefore finds meaning primarily in his work, is forced to retire, he cannot cope. The woman whose principal sense of identity is tied up in her husband cannot cope when she finds out he has been having an affair. The man who learned to rarely express his feelings feels trapped in a situation that can be improved only if he expresses himself openly.

4. *The individual sees no way of changing the rules about how he or she must act and so feels trapped and helpless to resolve the problem.* Because the unconscious decisions of the "right way" to be form a significant part of their identity, these people may not see that change is possible or may even feel that to change significantly is to lose their identity. Most of our patients acknowledge that there was a time prior to the onset of their illness when they felt helpless, unable to solve or control problems in their lives, and found themselves "giving up."

They saw themselves as "victims"—months before the onset of cancer—because they no longer felt capable of altering their lives in ways that would resolve their problems or reduce their stresses. Life happened to them; they did not control it. They were acted upon rather than actors. The continued stresses were final proof to them that time and further developments would not improve their lot.

5. *The individual puts distance between himself or herself and the problem, becoming static, unchanging, rigid.* Once there is no hope, then the individual is just "running in place," never expecting to go anywhere. On the surface he or she may seem to be coping with life, but internally life seems to hold no further meaning, except in maintaining the conventions. Serious illness or death represents a solution, an exit, or a postponement of the problem.

Although many of our patients remember this thought sequence, others are not consciously aware of it. Most, however, will recall having had feelings of helplessness or hopelessness some months prior to the onset of the disease. This process does not *cause* cancer, rather, it *permits* cancer to develop.

It is this giving–up on life that plays a role in interfering with the immune system and may, through changes in hormonal balance, lead to an increase in the production of abnormal cells. Physically, it creates a climate that is right for the development of cancer.

The crucial point to remember is that all of us create the *meaning* of events in our lives. The individual who assumes the victim stance *participates* by assigning meanings to life events that prove there is no hope. Each of us *chooses*—although not always at a conscious level—how we are going to react. The intensity of the stress is determined by the meaning we assign to it and the rules we have established for how we will cope with stress.

In outlining this process it is not our intention to make anyone feel guilty or frightened—that would only make matters worse. Instead, we hope that if we can see ourself in this psychological process, we will recognize it as a call to action and make changes in our lives. Since emotional states contribute to illness, they can also contribute to health. By acknowledging our own participation in the onset of the disease, we acknowledge our power to participate in regaining our health and we have also taken the first step toward getting well again.

GETTING WELL AGAIN

We have just described the psychological steps we have identified and observed in a patient's becoming ill. It's important to appreciate that many of these steps occur unconsciously, without the patient's awareness that he or she was even participating. The whole purpose of explaining the psychological steps in the spiral toward illness is to build a basis from which the patient can proceed to the steps in a spiral toward recovery.

By becoming aware of the spiral that occurred in the development of their own illness, many of our patients take the first step in altering its direction. Then, by changing attitudes and behavior, they can tip the scales in the direction of health.

We have observed four psychological steps that occur in the upward spiral of recovery:

1. *With the diagnosis of a life–threatening illness, the individual gains a new perspective on his or her problems.* Many of the rules by which an individual lives suddenly seem petty and insignificant in the face of death. In effect, the threat gives the individual permission to act in ways that did not seem permissible before. Held–in anger and hostility can now be expressed; assertive behavior is now allowed. Illness permits the person to say no.

2. *The individual makes a decision to alter behavior, to be a different kind of person.* Because the illness often suspends the rules, suddenly there are options. As behaviors change, apparently unresolvable conflicts may show signs of resolution. The individual begins to see that it is within his or her power to solve or cope with problems. He also discovers that life did not end when old rules were broken and that changes in behavior did not result in loss of identity. Thus there is more freedom to act and more resources with which to live. Depression often lifts when repressed feelings have been released and increased psychological energy is available.

Based on these new experiences, the individual makes a decision to be a different kind of person; the disease serves as permission to change.

3. *Physical processes in the body respond to the feelings of hope and the renewed desire to live, creating a reinforcing cycle with the new mental state.* The renewed hope and desire to live initiate physical processes that result in improved health. Since mind, body, and emotions act as a system, changes in the psychological state result in changes in the physical state. This is a continuing cycle, with an improved physical state bringing renewed hope in life and with renewed hope bringing additional physical improvement.

In most cases, this process has its ups and downs. Patients may do very well physically until their renewed physical health brings them face–to–face with one of their areas of psychological conflict. If one of the conflicts has had to do with a job, for example, the physical disability associated with the illness may have temporarily removed the conflict because the individual was unable to work. With physical health restored, however, the patient may be facing again the stressful life situations. Even with renewed hope and a different perception of self and the problems, these are usually difficult times. There may be temporary physical setbacks until the patient again feels confident enough to cope with the situation.

4. *The recovered patient is "weller than well."* Karl Menninger, founder of the Menninger Clinic, describes patients who have recovered from bouts with mental illness as frequently being "weller than well," meaning that the state of emotional health to which they have been restored is in fact superior to what they had considered "well" before their illness. Much the same observation applies to patients who have actively participated in recovery from cancer. They have a psychological strength, a positive self–concept, a sense of control over their lives that clearly represent an improved level of psychological devel-

opment. Many patients who have been active in their recovery have a positively altered stance toward life, expecting things will go well—victims no more.

REFERENCES

1. Galen. *De tumoribus* [About tumors].
2. Gendron, D. *Enquiries into nature, knowledge, and cure of cancers.* London, 1701.
3. Burrows, J. *A practical essay on cancer.* London, 1783.
4. Bernard, C. *Experimental medicine.* 1865.
5. Paget, J. *Surgical pathology* (2nd ed.). London: Longman's Green, 1870.
6. Snow, H. *Cancer and the cancer process.* London: J. & A. Churchill, 1893.
7. Achterberg, J., Simonton, O.C., & Matthews-Simonton, S. *Stress, psychological factors, and cancer.* Fort Worth: New Medicine Press, 1976.
8. Evans, E. *A psychological study of cancer.* New York: Dodd, Mead & Company, 1926.
9. LeShan, L.L. *You can fight for your life.* New York: M. Evans & Company, 1977.
10. LeShan, L.L. An emotional life history pattern associated with neoplastic disease. *Annals of the New York Academy of Sciences,* 1966, *125,* 780–793.
11. Thomas, C.B., & Duszynski, D.R. Closeness to parents and the family constellation in a prospective study of five disease states: Suicide, mental illness, malignant tumor, hypertension, and coronary heart disease. *The Johns Hopkins Medical Journal,* 1974, *134,* 251–270.
12. Schmale, A.H., & Iker, H. Hopelessness as a predictor of cervical cancer. *Social Science and Medicine,* 1971, *5,* 95–100.
13. Greene, W.A., Jr. The psychosocial setting of the development of leukemia and lymphoma. *Annals of the New York Academy of Sciences,* 1966, *125,* 794–801.
14. Kissen, D.M. The significance of personality in lung cancer in men. *Annals of the New York Academy of Sciences,* 1966, *125,* 933–945.
15. Blumberg, E.M., West, P.M., & Ellis, F.W. A possible relationship between psychological factors and human cancer. *Psychosomatic Medicine,* 1954, *16,* (4), 276–286.
16. Klopfer, B. Psychological variables in human cancer. *Journal of Projective Techniques,* 1957, *21,* 331–340.
17. Green, E. & Green, A. *Beyond biofeedback.* New York: Delacorte, 1977.
18. Simonton, O.C., Matthews–Simonton, S., & Creighton, J. *Getting well again.* Los Angeles: J. P. Tarcher, Inc., 1978.

Part V

THE HEALING CONNECTION

Health promotion, patient education, and practitioner change are indispensable parts of integral medicine. The first establishes the larger health–care context of which treatment of illness is but part. Educated patients and a cooperative relationship between practitioners and the consumers of health care forms the necessary precondition for health promotion. Finally, a more integrated holistic approach to health care can come about only if its practitioners are willing and able to meet the changing needs of those who come to them for help.

The three chapters in this section present variations on the themes of patient education, health promotion, and practitioner change. In Chapter 13 Dennis Jaffe describes the kind of sensitive approach to behavioral counseling and education that any clinician might utilize in his or her therapeutic work.

Paul Brenner, M.D., a 47–year–old physician who left the clinical practice of obstetrics and gynecology to assist people in assuming responsibility for their own health care, discusses in Chapter 14 the evolutionary process of an integrally oriented doctor. He is the author of *Health is a Question of Balance* (DeVorss Press, 1980) and numerous scientific articles. Dr. Brenner is an assistant clinical professor of Reproductive Medicine at the University of California at San Diego, and a member of the Executive Council of the Center for Integral Medicine.

John Travis, a physician trained in preventive medicine, explores the concept of wellness in Chapter 15. Dr. Travis believes that the emphasis in medical education on pathological functioning has limited the utility of most physicians. Though they may be able to treat and cure some diseases, they are unable to help their patients to become aware of and to act to change the habits of thought and behavior which keep them from feeling completely well. He suggests that some physicians continue to be trained for curative medicine while others be trained to promote wellness.

John Travis, M.D., M.P.H., studied at Tufts University School of Medicine in Boston and completed a residency in Preventive Medicine at Johns Hopkins. He set aside practicing medicine in favor of helping people to restructure their lifestyle so that they can take full responsibility for their health. He was founder and Director of the Wellness Resource Center in Mill Valley, California, now known as Wellness Associates.

Chapter 12

SELF–MANAGEMENT AND BEHAVIORAL MEDICINE: SEIZING CONTROL OF SELF–DEFEATING BEHAVIOR

Dennis T. Jaffe, Ph.D.

Most individuals do not worry about their health until they lose it. Uncertain attempts at healthy living may be thwarted by the temptations of a culture whose economy depends on high production and high consumption . . . Facing the insufferable insult of extinction with the years, and knowing how we might improve our health, we still don't do much about it . . .

Prevention of disease means forsaking the bad habits which many people enjoy—overeating, too much drinking, taking pills, staying up at night, engaging in promiscuous sex, driving too fast, and smoking cigarettes—or, put another way, it means doing things which require special effort—exercising regularly, going to the dentist, practicing contraception, ensuring harmonious family life, submitting to screening examinations. The idea of individual responsibility flies in the face of American history which has seen a people steadfastly sanctifying individual freedom while progressively narrowing it through the development of a beneficient state . . . The cost of sloth, gluttony, alcoholic intemperance, reckless driving, sexual frenzy, and smoking is now a national, and not an individual, responsibility . . . I believe the idea of a "right" to health should be replaced by the idea of an individual moral obligation to preserve one's health—a public duty if you will.

—John Knowles
"The Responsibility of the Individual"
Daedalus, Winter, 1977, p. 59.

BEHAVIOR CHANGE AS A MEDICAL PROBLEM

The changes demanded of patients in treatment fall in two rough categories. The first has been labeled "treatment," "treatment adherence," or "compliance." Activities that the patient has to carry out in the treatment process include taking medication regularly, at the appropriate times and as long as necessary; attending follow–up appointments; attending to personal hygiene and precautions during the active phase of disease and convalescence if medically necessary. Barry Blackwell[1] has noted that only about one–half of all physicians' recommendations for treatment are carried out. For example, patients medicate themselves at will, and often act as if they did not want to get well. Recent research has focused on psychological methods to increase adherence and has led to a series of programmatic recommendations to physicians concerning how to package and present treatment plans to maximize the probability that they will be carried out.

The second mode of patient change consists of alterations in patterns of self–destructive or dangerous habits which will or may affect future health. Physicians routinely admonish patients to slow down, relax more, get proper rest, stop smoking, exercise, and alter their dietary patterns. But they often provide little active guidance in exactly how to achieve these massive changes. Increasingly, physicians have included self–care, stress management, weight control, smoking reduction and health promotion in their practice. They have devised strategies to help their patients create programs for change.

Increasing adherence and altering health–threatening behavior demand a change in the roles and modes of activity of both the patient and the physician. Both parties have an expanded set of responsibilities and can be expected to do more and to be more involved with each other. The patient, no longer a passive recipient of treatment, has certain specific tasks and responsibilities to fulfill in order to make the treatment work. Similarly, the physician has to move out of his technical role to become more of an educator, counselor, guide, and support person. If he or she does not choose to do so, then someone else must be delegated responsibility for these tasks. Patient and physician, along with allied health professionals, must become partners in the treatment process.

Taking this new role seriously places an additional burden on the physician. In the more traditional medical role, the physician dispensed treatment and advice. While it remains the patient's responsibility to heed advice and to commit himself to the full change process demanded of comprehensive treatment, the physician now has a variety of psychological methods—behavior modification, mental imagery, hypnosis—to help accomplish the tasks of education, persuasion, motivation, commitment, and behavior change. It is important for the health–care professional to make use of these techniques to help patients implement the regimens they advise; to substitute cooperative care and self–management for simple prescription.

To help physicians change their patients' behavior and to promote more healthy lifestyles, I created the Learning for Health program in Los Angeles. My aim is to provide psychological resources to physicians and to aid patients in the difficult, painful, and confusing process of change which accompanies the therapy of chronic illness and behavior disorders. While the physician has the responsibility for medical treatment, my role is primarily in the areas of psychological support and behavioral change. Along with the patient and physician, I then become a third partner in the comprehensive health team. This paper focuses on the process of change as part of medical treatment.

A Case Study—Lynn:
The Many Facets
of a Weight–control Program

Lynn, a 40–year–old married woman, had been gaining weight gradually for 15 years. She entered Learning for Health after receiving a diagnosis of "dangerously high blood pressure." I learned that she had lost several hundred pounds over the years on various crash diets and at health spas but had always gained it back. Now, when a serious medical complication ensued—in part because of her eating habits—she was frightened enough to try making a lasting change. She was willing to commit herself to a special diet—low in cholesterol, salt and calories—that was critical to lowering her blood pressure.

As do many people, Lynn ate when she was under stress. Her parents had inadvertently taught her that rich and flavorful food was a great and satisfying gift. She felt devoid of all "will power" to avoid food. Additionally, her body had never felt good to her; she had always perceived herself as fat and ugly. Except for finely defined face and hands, her image of herself was round and featureless. Her sensitivity to most sensation and movement was low; physical exercise was pure drudgery to her.

Working together, we began with a period of self–observation, aimed at making her aware of habits, feelings, and behavior patterns related to food and health. She kept a daily log of what she ate, when she ate, where she ate, how she felt before and after meals, her daily exercise regimens, and the stressful events of each day. By the end of the first week of structured, written self–observation, she was anxious and depressed at her inability to curb her eating. She felt "bad" and considered her plight hopeless.

In order to initiate change, a person needs to experience at least some small degree of success that demonstrates how his or her habits and life can be successfully changed. With this principle in mind, I decided that Lynn's first task should be to increase her body awareness and control over stress, both of which contributed indirectly to her eating.

These tasks are relatively easy and feel good. I reasoned that some success in them might increase her motivation to take on the more difficult tasks which would follow. Because she had such a long history of failure at changing eating patterns, I felt that her food intake should be approached only after she successfully made other changes.

With the help of a cassette, I taught Lynn an exercise in progressive relaxation. I suggested that she try to relax during the most stressful periods of the day, particularly at those times when she habitually ate. My goal was to teach her a new response to stress—to susbtitute the pleasant habit of relaxation of her self–destructive and ineffectual eating.

At the same time, I started Lynn on an exercise program designed to help her find ways to use her body that were easy, pleasant, and easily assimilable into her lifestyle. She enjoyed swimming and bicycle riding with a friend, as I suggested, to reinforce her own commitment to exercise. Her habitual morning coffee and rolls were replaced by swimming and bike riding. After only two weeks, she felt better physically, more confident, more alive, and less stressed. Incidentally, during this period, I had instructed her to eat what she wanted and not to weigh herself. I did not want her focus to be on eating or on weight control.

Next we began to explore Lynn's eating patterns. Because Lynn was responsible for preparing her family's meals as well as her own, this phase of the program needed the cooperation and participation of her household members, particularly her husband. He was healthy and slim, and not particularly concerned about his wife's weight. He kidded her about her dieting and always asked for large meals. Her teenage sons, active in athletics, also liked high–calorie meat and carbohydrate foods. Though it caused them some discomfort, Lynn's family agreed to help her change because they were concerned enough about her health to make some sacrifices to their palate.

Lynn agreed to serve herself smaller portions of food, to eat more slowly, and to eliminate dessert. Everyone in the family stopped drinking caffeinated coffee and her husband, eager to support her efforts at self–care, began to give her massages.

The changes in family meals helped, but they were not the major problem. Her most destructive eating occurred primarily when she was home alone. When anxious, bored, or under stress, she would wolf down the junk food kept in the larder.

Accordingly, the next stage of Lynn's behavioral change program consisted of three steps. The first was to restructure her environment. Many foods were eliminated from her shopping list. Lynn consciously began to avoid the kitchen. Conversations about food and eating (and especially about Lynn's diet) were curtailed in the family. When the temptation to eat became strong, she was instructed to do something else besides eat—walk out of the house, call someone on the phone, or simply remind herself of her commitment to change and its positive consequences.

The second aspect of Lynn's change program was an exploration of the deepest thoughts, beliefs and feelings that she associated with food, weight, health, and her body. In therapeutic sessions with me, for example, Lynn discovered that she associated thinness with an attractiveness and sexuality that made her uneasy. Later, as she became aware of how she used food as a self–reward, she began to develop a new belief system. Now she felt she would reward herself by not eating. At her own instruction, she regularly reminded herself how much better she felt when she limited her food intake.

Finally, Lynn began to examine her positive, future goals. Concluding that eating had concealed a sense of inner emptiness and had been a substitute for meaningful companionship, she began to search for a career and made some long–needed changes in her marriage.

Lynn lost weight steadily for a year. She joined a health–support group in which other people were also making major life changes. Her blood pressure decreased, and, consequently, she required less medication and suffered fewer unpleasant side effects. She felt better and became more optimistic about her future.

Before Lynn's story is ended, some of the things that she did not do should be noted. She did not weigh herself regularly, or become obsessed about whether she was gaining or losing weight. Nor did she adhere to a strict diet or count calories. Instead, she altered her basic attitudes, patterns, and behavior toward food, exercise, her body, and herself. Food became less important as other aspects of her life took its place. Within a year, her goal of permanently altering her health–threatening behavior was accomplished.

THE FIVE STAGES OF SELF–MANAGEMENT

Prior to dramatically changing her life, Lynn shared a problem with a majority of Americans—an automatic, unconscious eating behavior which had gradually evolved into a health hazard. Some studies indicate that perhaps 90 percent of Americans will die prematurely from "diseases of civilization" that stem, directly or indirectly, from their relationship to food, exercise and the environment.[2] Ironically, many people are aware of the risks they face. Many have, in fact, unsuccessfully tried diets and a succession of exercise programs.

Why do people find it so difficult to adhere to vitally important efforts at self–control? One factor certainly is the short–term pleasure of inappropriate behavior, and the delayed nature of its negative consequences. Many people prefer to deal with life like gamblers, playing the odds that they won't contract heart disease or cancer. Our culture's denial of mortality, and our refusal to realize the body's limits, promotes this attitude. Besides, it is difficult to renounce what everyone else seems to enjoy.

Even so, people's bodies eventually tell them that change is needed. They begin to feel the effects of unhealthy behavior and consequently resolve to change eating and smoking habits, to treat their bodies better. Some resolve to channel their energy against the strong current of habits and desires. Yet, no matter how hard they try, they regress to old ways. Attempting to change habits through will is similar to trying to relax or fall asleep by active force. Will alone is ineffective against the power of deeply ingrained unconscious habits. In such situations people must apply principles of learning and behavior change. Rather than trying to force change on his or her patients, a health professional can help them first to understand and simplify the process of change, then to proceed in small steps—with a guide or helper—or in a small group, on a complete and effective program of behavior change.

What follows is an outline of the procedure I use to help people change self–destructive habits and behavior patterns. Though most of the illustrations are drawn from Lynn's case history, the method is as applicable to other habits and to the treatment of chronic pain as it is to weight control. The thrust of the entire program is the elimination of factors that promote negative health habits and reinforcement of positive behaviors.

There are five stages in my program to reverse dysfunctional habits of behavior:

> Self–observation—becoming aware of the nature of the habit and the context in which it occurs.
>
> Mobilization of "motivation"—the energy and commitment that carry a person through the change process.
>
> Creation of a change strategy and a contract for specific action.
>
> Practice of alternate responses to situations that usually lead one to respond habitually and the creation of newer, more adaptive habits.
>
> Establishment of a network of people to support the new, more adaptive habits.

This sequence can be used to alter almost any type of negative habit, from sexual impotency, obesity, shyness, and destructive marital conflicts to stress symptoms, headaches, bedwetting, back pain, and insomnia. Each of these habits or symptoms has been inadvertently learned. Treatment consists of modifying the environment so that it demands or supports different behaviors.

Let us consider each stage in more detail. The first stage involves a careful study of the habit, a study that requires a week to a month of self–observation to discover exactly when, where and under what circumstances the habit evolved. I suggest that the patient begin by carrying a sheet of paper and, as Lynn did, noting when certain types of habits or feelings appear. Each day an inventory is made of the kinds of responses, emotions and situations associated with the problem.

For example, when people like Lynn want to change their eating habits, I ask them to chart each bite of food they take, how they eat it, where they eat it, and what they were doing and feeling at the time and afterwards. Patients who have headaches or other pain problems chart the degree of their discomfort or stress at hourly intervals on a scale of 0 to 5, what they are doing and feeling at the time pain comes and how they dealt with it—including whether or not they take medication. This hourly chart makes a person aware, often for the first time, of how prevalent and habitual pain or stress is in his or her life. Clear–cut patterns also emerge. For instance, some people have colds or headaches only on weekends and holidays.

One woman I treated suffered migraine headaches almost weekly for many years. Through the inventory she discovered that her head-aches typically occurred a few hours after doing something she didn't want to do, or after she had been angry. I then asked her to note in her daily inventory anything she did during the day that made her furious, or that she disliked doing. The next time we met, she told me she ran out of paper writing it all down. This exercise helped her finally to see how pervasive her anger was and to correct its frustrated expression.

Once the individual becomes aware of the problem, he can enter the second stage—the search for "motivation," the energy to carry out the change process. Motivation is usually thought of as an internal force that prompts us to do or not to do various things. But behavioral psychologists perceive motivation or "will power" as simply the end result of a number of internal and external factors, many of which are in conflict with one another. If the sum total is positive, we do something, if not, we don't.

When a person speaks of finding, or having, motivation, what is probably meant is creating enough incentives or eliminating enough obstacles to accomplish a specific goal. For example, if one's salary were dependent on observing proper health habits, or if sugar, salt, tobacco, alcohol and food additives were illegal drugs entailing severe punishments for their possession, most people would revise their con-sumption to match these disincentives. But we live in a world where advertisements, fast–food restaurants, convenience foods, and abun-dance continually reinforce unhealthy habits. Against this environ-mental barrage of reinforcements we must learn to motivate ourselves to be healthier.

As the first step in building positive motivation, I ask patients to list as many reasons as they can for each of their bad habits. The list should contain all the environmental factors that tempt or persuade them to keep the habit, including people, situations, and feelings. It also might include the subtle benefits obtained from the bad habits.

During illness, for instance, people often receive considerable nurturing, care, and help from others. It may be hard to give up back pain—and the accompanying attention—when it means going back to a dreary job.

Next, patients are asked to compile another list (usually shorter) of reasons to change. For many people, the first item on the list is, "The doctor said I had to." When a person actually experiences the consequences of a bad habbit—shortness of breath, difficulty walking, continual pain, etc.—these reasons become strong incentives to change.

It is not uncommon to feel a sense of loss in abandoning a pleasurable habit. Therefore, patients need to make a final list in which they devise a strategy for obtaining each of the benefits of their bad habits without acting destructively. For example, they might ask directly for attention instead of complaining about their pain.

The third stage of the program is critical. It involves examining the lists of positive and negative incentives and designing a program for change. Management psychologist Chris Argyris[3] has conducted research which shows that people are more likely to carry out a change program if they have helped select their own change goals and the particular approaches used to achieve them. This is especially true if they are the object of the change. Many programs for change fail because goals are imposed and not tailored to and shared with the individual who is to change.

The physician and patient must work together to create the program for change. This program may involve one master plan and may include small weekly or monthly steps and goals that specify particular changes. Certainly, the goals must be clear and specific. Rather than striving "to lose weight" one might do better aiming toward "losing thirty–five pounds within six months by modifying eating behavior and adopting a vigorous exercise program." The reasons and incentives for the goals, as well as the obstacles and deterrents, should be specified. This program should be in writing, signed by the patient and his or her physician—and, perhaps, a family member or close friend who will help in the program. It is also helpful to incorporate specific rewards. For example, after achieving his goals for the week, a patient might do something that he likes or treats himself to something special. And it is essential that this contract, like any good contract, be concrete, realistic and specific.

The fourth stage of the change program involves adopting newer and healthier habits. Role playing—or actually trying out new responses in make-believe situations—can be helpful in initially learning new habits. For instance, patients can practice saying "no," or even leaving the table, when they are offered food, when others smoke, or when they feel angry. They can vicariously experience the types of situations that give them trouble and create new responses to prepare themselves for the time when the situation actually arises. At first new habits are difficult to learn. It is not easy to learn to wake up forty minutes earlier to jog, or to avoid the kitchen. But in time new habits become automatic and easy.

In the final stage of altering dysfunctional habits, the physician or therapists make sure that a patient has continuing support for the new responses. Since the patient's customary environment has usually not been supportive of healthy behavior, a group will probably need to be actively recruited—e.g., the family—to offer such support. Actually, it is easier for an entire family (or couple) than for an individual to diet or stop smoking, or to adopt an exercise or relaxation regimen. A family whose members work together to change behavior and have fun doing it, praising and coaxing each other along the way, is the most effective vehicle for change. Such an environment creates its own motivation.

Beyond the family, the best way to support new behavior is through a self–help group of men and women with the same problem. The self–help movement has a long and distinguished history of aiding individuals to change behavior, yet, thus far, few physicians have made use of these groups as parts of their programs.[45] One of the oldest and most effective of these programs is Alcoholics Anonymous, founded and run entirely by exalcoholics. AA had developed one of the few successful ways of persuading people to stop drinking. In recent years, other self–help groups have been formed to address themselves to almost every type of difficulty and illness. Weight Watchers is the best known, but there are hundreds of others, including postmastectomy, poststroke, hypertension groups, and an organization for people with cancer and other terminal illnesses called "Make Today Count."

In adjusting to chronic illness, or searching for lasting change of a health–threatening behavior, a small group is more likely to be useful than a single physician. By exchanging agreements or commitments with other people rather than a physician, and by keeping in contact with these men and women when there is difficulty in adhering to the contract, patients can make use of a powerful and readily available source of help. Members of those groups strongly value positive, health–supporting behavior and understand the difficulties a patient faces. Thus they can provide the support for adaptation and change missing from the normal environment.

This kind of program for modifying health–threatening behavior demands greater involvement and more time investment in patient care than physicians have been accustomed to offering. However, as Americans suffer in greater numbers from chronic and from habit–caused illnesses which are, in theory, preventable, such programs become increasingly necessary. Where changes in habits and behavior are essential to patient health, methods for bringing about behavioral change will become more central to medical practice. Finally, as family physicians become more concerned with promoting health of the entire family, rather than treating their diseases, education and self–care programs will become as much a part of routine treatment as the annual check up.

REFERENCES

1. Blackwell, B., Treatment adherence. *British Journal of Psychiatry*, 1976, 129, 513–531.
2. Knowles, J., The responsibility of the individual. *Daedalus*, 1977, *106*, 57–80.
3. Agryris, C., *Interpersonal competance and organizational effectiveness*. Homewood, Illinois: Irwin & Dorsey, 1962.
4. Katz, A., & Bender, E., *The strength in U.S.: Self–help groups and the modern world*. New York: Viewpoints, 1976.
5. Levin, L.S., Katz, A.H., & Holst, E. *Self–care: Lay initiatives in health*. New York: Prodist, Neale Watson Academic Publications, 1976.

Chapter 13

A PERSONAL TRAJECTORY

Paul Brenner, M.D.

After 11 years in the private practice of obstetrics and gynecology, I left traditional medicine and entered the field of health maintenance, sharing thoughts of diet, exercise, meditation, and do–it–yourself health techniques with groups of people. As an introduction, I'd like briefly to share some of the events in my life that led to this change in my medical career. The inciting motivation was the Women's Movement of the late sixties which targeted gynecologists for not being responsive to the needs of women, and more importantly for not providing their patients with medical and health information.

At about this time, I first realized that the withholding of information from a patient laid the basis for the uneasiness and inequality that frustrates so much medical care. It became clear to me that I was involved not only in a patient's medical problem, but in their social and family life. Postoperative questions such as "Could I drive to Los Angeles today?" or "When can I start making love with my husband?" should be anticipated prior to discharge. By waiting for such questions to be asked, the patient is placed in a dependent and thus subservient role. The Women's Movement speaks to the individual rights of all human beings: to be treated as equals and to be educated to the level of the teacher.

In 1971 I established a free clinic in San Diego, showing "street people" how to do adequate physical examination and simple laboratory tests. The ease with which they learned these skills forced me to question the time and effort that went into my own training. I soon appreciated that by sharing my knowledge, I could help patients take responsibility for their own health; by delegating certain functions to them, I could use my mind and my training with greater certainty.

In 1972 I attended an acupuncture symposium at Stanford University. Although the therapeutic triumphs attributed to this ancient form of healing seemed impossible, I was intrigued enough to study further with Dr. Felix Mann in London and Dr. Shen Lee in Taiwan. Upon returning to San Diego, I asked two medical students to evaluate various skin areas for the points of decreased resistance which were supposed to characterize acupuncture points. In four hours, they plotted an acupuncture chart that was identical to the one published 2500 years before Christ in the *Yellow Emperor's Classic of Internal Medicine.*

I began to perform acupuncture on willing patients, continuing to apply my modern, Western scientific paradigms to this ancient Eastern form of healing. The model, however, did not fit. It eventually occurred to me that what I had learned in medical school was based on models that predicted results which fit within two standard deviations. My experience with acupuncture, if nothing else, led me to question my entire reality system.

In order to evaluate the placebo effect of acupuncture, I experimented on various animals. If, indeed, this healing art did work, then this would stand as scientific proof to my colleagues. To my amazement and joy results with animals far exceeded those that were achieved with my patients.

My great desire for this therapeutic procedure to work led me to another level of questioning the success with acupuncture. Was it possible that my own belief systems were effecting cures? If that were the case, could scientists perhaps affect the results that "unbiasedly" appeared in the test tube and were confirmed by double–blind studies? When I suggested to my fellow physicians that the strength of my convictions, not the efficacy of acupuncture, might explain my success, they suddenly jumped to accept acupuncture as a viable veterinary therapy. It was far more believable than healing through a directed belief and a far better procedure for animals than humans. One does not have to know why something works on animals.

These results led me to further my studies in placebo research and in learning and memory mechanisms. If placebo works 35 percent of the time, as most studies show, why not study the individuals with whom it works, learn how they make use of the placebo, and apply the technique to the 65 percent who seem to need conventional medicine?

In 1974 I experienced the expansiveness and plasticity of the mind through personal work in isolation tanks. In such an environment, all sensory input is eliminated and content is internally orchestrated. I began to explore my own consciousness, finding memory loops, and even apparitions within my own brain that were spontaneously recalled. I attempted to meditate in the watery isolation but found it impossible; without an appreciation of my five senses I was no more than mind energy. I was, in fact, the meditation. In the tank, as there were no sensory perceptions, I could not create any experiences; I was a totality of all my experiences.

I then devised a form of meditation and practiced it outside the tank. I learned that in the quietness of meditation one can hear; the intuition that evolves following this silence, if applied, then serves as a major source of creativity and telepathy. This was followed by a brief instruction by Dr. Evarts Loomis in the importance of diet, fasting, homeopathy, and, more importantly, Walt Whitman. I soon realized that the works of Wheeler and Mehro, Heisenberg, and Einstein were not in any way different from the philosophical concepts of Lao Tsu, Tarthang Tulku, and Alice Bailey. Modern post–Einsteinian physics and ancient mystics sounded so much alike that it seemed science served only to validate the intuitive knowledge of esoterism. I then studied with various types of "healers," accepting their nontraditional treatments as valid therapeutic modalities for such clients as sought them out.

In an effort to extend and act upon the sense of connectedness I had begun to feel immediately following the first earthquakes in Guatemala, I felt compelled to assist the people in that country. My experiences taught me that the degree of sadness, suffering, and grief among the Guatemalans appeared to be directly proportional to the proximity of the people to the metropolitan areas. Those who lived closer to the metropolitan areas could find little solace within themselves, having exchanged for personal possessions any sense of personal harmony. I realized how many of us in the United States are also prisoners of our possessions, expectations, and, ultimately, our past; few of us live in a fluid state in the present. I soon appreciated that I received more than I gave.

Finally, in 1976, I left my practice, not because I did not love my work or feel that is was a valid form of healing, but because I was suffocating from the dependency that I had allowed my patients to have on me. I realized that my own need to be a doctor, to be depended on, were preventing individuals from accepting their own responsibility. On the other hand, patients willfully allowed this exploitation for their benefit. They abdicated their responsibility for their own health and well–being in order that they could devote themselves to anything else (work or a significant other) in life other than themselves. Perhaps accepting responsibility for themselves was too frightening. The doctor–patient relationship seemed a symbiotic, yet unholy alliance in which participants in the game seek ego–strength from without rather than from within themselves.

The two snakes entwining the staff of Hermes represent a more ideal doctor–patient relationship—one of equality at each level of ascendance. If the Western physician continues to assume complete responsibility for patients, the snakes, instead of ascending, will coil and strike and so consume themselves. The new physician must be a provider–teacher who will assist individuals in assuming responsibility for themselves. I would like to suggest that this new physician operate on a new medical paradigm, one based on philosophy and physics. In the future healing will be a cocreative process shared by the healer and the healed. In such a mode, the person to be healed also teaches and heals the physician.

HEALTH AND ILLNESS

In my book, *Health is a Question of Balance,* health is described as a balance between hyper and hypo states of illness, polarized states of disease, homeostasis. In another sense, the opposite of a given disease is not health but another disease, while at the midpoint of the continuum a constant vacillation exists between health and "dishealth." This conforms to the Taoist principle that the only constant is change. If dishealth (i.e., the transient loss of health) is stabilized over prolonged periods of time, then illness manifests. The mutability of health to disease (illness) and vice versa depends on a definite quantum of dishealth.

For example, if one considers 130/90 to be the upper limit of normal blood pressure and 140/100 to be frank hypertension, then a minimal increment in dishealth is associated with a major change in the health state; yet, a minimal amount of therapy will not reverse the process. The quantity of energy in the form of therapy needed to reverse this state may be equivalent to the amount of dishealth utilized in the process of raising the blood pressure from 100/70 to 140/100, not from 130/90 to 140/100. Once this state is established, a minimal increment of illness requires a disproportionate quantum of therapy to reverse the state. Therefore, as the blood pressure approaches 150/100, the amount of therapy needed to achieve health may triple—or all therapy may become ineffective. If there is not enough energy to sustain the illness or to reverse the process—then death occurs.

In this paradigm, the upper or lower limit of normal is abnormal. Adherence to this paradigm requires physicians to be trained in health maintenance through understanding specific individuals in their unique environments. It demands that they be knowledgeable enough to prescribe the correct amounts of diet, exercise, or mind games (i.e., meditation, imagery, journal keeping, etc.) to maintain that individual's self–health. A normal range must be individualized for the specific patient, and, as he or she deviates from the unique norm, therapy should be initiated before disease becomes manifest.

The major factor in overcoming the inertia of health and setting a path for dishealth is stress, that invisible ingredient in the environment whose presence we occasionally acknowledge, which, unless stabilized, can alter our physical state. As in Brownian movement (The Random Movement of Suspended Particles), there are invisible factors in our environment that are constantly bombarding us and displacing us from our apparent normal path. In a Zen sense, this is the reason for our impermanence. If the milieu is not changed and the agitation continues, then displacement is towards disease, that is, away from the center—health. Since social stress is not in the spectrum of human visibility, it has an insidious effect, usually not being perceived until a definite quantity has caused an effect, that is, pain, illness, or suffering.

The quantum of stress needed to produce a given effect is variable for different individuals, but for any given individual there is a specific amount of stress or sum of varied stresses over a period of time which will lead to frank disease (or distress). Brownian movement provides a useful analogy: As one increases the viscosity (stability) of the environment, one will effectively decrease the agitation (stress). The converse is also true: Some people are too stuck in an unhealthy non-fluid fixed environment and need to be agitated to create change and restore health. In a sense these latter are living in a vacuum which does not provide either nourishment for growth or room for change.

Agitation *per se* is not good or bad; as the Taoists would suggest, it is relative. Stress is our society tends to have a negative connotation, but even positive events as vacation and retirement are stressful situations. The number of acute coronaries seen in emergency rooms in the vacation areas of the United States attests to this statement. Sudden, dynamic, unresolved stress establishes the culture medium on which the germ theory has been validated, while fluidity and balance are the media of unexplained natural resistance and health.

As a gynecologist, I was impressed by the numbers of vaginal infections that naval fliers' wives incurred during the stressful weeks before and after their husbands left for air–carrier maneuvers. There is no question that offending organisms such as trichomonads or monilia were present on microscopic examination—but why did the infection manifest only under the stress of a husband leaving, or at the joy of his return? The same circumstances were associated with an increased incidence of menometrorrhagia and pregnancy–related complications.

Stress is anything that alters the course of human events. It is essential for creative transformation, movement, and change. In many ways, stress can be equated with the Zen concept of suffering. If understood, it can serve as a prime mover in reaching new goals; if not appreciated, it may be the initiator of dishealth. It is all a question of balance. Metaphorically speaking, it can be likened to a sailboat. The wind provides momentum. As the velocity of the wind increases, the boat is more likely to reach its destination. However, as the wind approaches gale force the aware sailor knows he or she must take down the sail, allow the wind to pass the mast, and await the termination of the storm before beginning the journey home.

Therefore the physician's role is not simply to look at pathology (the end result of a chain of discernible causes) but to gain insight into environments that modify health, the stage upon which the pathology is played out. If I am concerned with psychosomatic illness, why shouldn't I explore the conditions necessary for psychosomatic health?

Another factor to consider is the expectations of the patient and therapist concerning the disease state. As a gravitational field alters electromagnetic waves, so do one's weighted expectations alter one's path and belief of what is. Medical information based on statistical phenomena is too often presented as inexorable fact, serving to reinforce one's expectations and affecting individual outcome.

If the patient realizes that there are holes within the medical structure which provide room for hope, he or she may transcend a belief system and possibly change the outcome of an illness. This is especially true for the cancer patient, for whom the diagnosis itself has a connotation of helplessness. In such cases, as Bertrand Russell states, "abstraction, difficult as it is, is the source of practical power." Physicians can no longer afford to deal in absolutes. They must provide space for hope.

EFFECT OF TIME

There is also the effect of time. If the interval between illness and therapy is short (i.e., acute) and if there is no extensive tissue damage, therapeutic results are usually good. For example, a professional athlete whose injury is treated immediately heals faster than can be accounted for by physical conditioning or motivation alone. If plotted mathmatically, this course will appear as a straight line conforming to Euclid, and the cause and effect laws of the twentieth-century medical paradigm.

On the other hand, if the disease process becomes chronic, as when a limb is traumatized before amputation, then the chance of a therapeutic triumph is lessened and the probability of phantom–limb pain increased. Time now has altered the apparent clarity of events and has affected the process of the disease. The physician must now take into account all the minievents which have been superimposed on the initial causality. The interval between events then takes on greater meaning than the events themselves, noncausal phenomena such as emotional rewards, drugs, and compensation affect the disease process. Recovery becomes difficult when the rewards of illness are greater than those received for health. When this occurs, the shortest distance between the event of illness and the event of seeking help is no longer a straight path based on the causality of Descartes but may be likened to the time–space warp of Riemann where "the shortest path between any two points follows the route that a body will take if left alone."

Although Paul Courderc's statement that the "interval between two events presents a more profound reality than the events themselves" was written in relationship to atomic physics, it applies also to understanding the individual human being. Events of man are not static but obey the laws of the space–time continuum. Space curvature is a result of a particle's path in a gravitational field. One's self–imposed expectations plus the bombardment of the expectations of others, plus the noncausal factors of the social environment, are the gravitational fields that one's path crosses. A case in point would be the patient with chronic low-back pain. The path between the herniation of a spinal disc in January and the event of seeing the physician a month or year later must pass through the new relationships the patient has with his family, work, sex, drug dependency, and the financial compensation provided by his health insurance. As in Einstein's general relativity theory, the dimension of time has filled the space between events with a multitude of microevents, the physician is forced to view illness as a plenum (a continually filled space in a field). The interval formed by chronic disease takes on more meaning than the etiology of the disease itself. Time has now affected causality. Cure depends on the unraveling of all events associated with the illness.

PHYSICIANS AS OBSERVER–PARTICIPANT

The physician, therefore, must become part of the field itself and can no longer remain solely in the role of an observer. In relation to quantum physics, John Wheeler suggests replacing the word "observer" by the word "participant." I feel that the role of the physician should be one of observer–participant. It is a role which is neither one of aloofness nor one of sympathy, but one of compassion. Heisenberg's uncertainty principle postulates that the observer affects his or her observations and that the closer one approaches an accurate figure for either the position or momentum of a particle, the less accurate becomes the figure for the other. By attempting to maintain the duality of observer–participant, the physician can approach a patient in a holistic sense. This means not only determining what happened and where it hurts, but also what was going on in the interim between the inciting insult and the "now moment" of the doctor–patient relationship. During this process, beliefs can be shared and goals established. The gate of acceptability between the healer and the healee can now open and, with shared knowledge, the healee becomes the healer. The physician and the patient trace the course of illness and recreate the engram (learning process) that continues to reinforce and stabilize the disease pattern. Physicians assist their clients in establishing new constructs that effectively block those recurring processes involved in illness.

Implicit in most anatomical and physiologic theories of learning is the concept that synaptic activation may lead to an increased effectiveness of the activation synapses and that sufficient repetition of an appropriate activation may lead to stabilization of this efficiency. This is dramatically demonstrated by the patient whose illness becomes a singular experience, one that cannot be shared. This patient may experience a contracted introspective existence wherein meditation upon the misfortune reinforces the despair, effectively recruiting synaptic representation of the illness and eventually stabilizing it. The disease then serves as static on a tape deck; the physician should attempt to remove the static so the previous normal tape of health can be heard. To accomplish this feat, the physician must find cause. Spinoza aptly that "suffering ceases to be suffering when one gets a clear, precise picture of it." I think that a complete picture of illness should incorporate not only the apparent cause but also the micro-events which habituate the illness. If this is not accomplished, therapy may be of only transient value, with either recurrence or a new disease process programmed by an inadequately treated engram. If, for example, any of the potentiating factors which were discussed in the case study of the patient with low–back pain was not resolved prior to therapy, that unresolved element might recreate the entire engram, causing reoccurrence of the pain in spite of the adequate therapy that the physician administers.

Lashley emphasized that any particular memory trace or engram has multiple representations throughout wide regions of the cortex. He concluded that any cortical neuron does not exclusively control one engram but that many neurons and synaptic junctions may relate to many engrams. Therefore, the recall of any one phenomenon in a memory process has the potential to recreate the entire engram or create a new one. This may explain why so many patients have one illness after another and are derogatorily referred to in medicine as malingerers. It would also account for the fact that chronic pain treated by various surgical procedures often reoccurs in sites other than that of its initial presentation. Simplistically stated, unless therapy relates to each element in the construct of the illness, it is not a complete therapy. This is reflected in Rosen's statement concerning the correctness of a physical theory in which he states "the correctness is judged by the degree of agreement between the conclusion of the theory and the human experience."

The proof of a cure does not necessarily rest solely on the resolution of the disease process. Cure is nothing more than an understanding of the process followed by a meaningful human change. Gurdjieff states that understanding is a balance between being and knowing. In this process of understanding, the disease ceases to be a disease, whether the process progresses or is reversed. If there is understanding and the patient now has direction and insight into his or her life, then this, in itself, is health. Health is the appreciation and acceptance of life. Individuals who live in the present or, as Orville Kelly suggests, make each day count, are not ill but are living out their unique design in their unique evolutionary processes. Conversely, people who cannot glean new meaning through the experience of illness and their insights into causality have not received correct or complete therapy, and they remain in a diseased physical state. All the elements of cause have not been determined, and recruitment within the engram of that illness maintains the illness.

Chapter 14

THE RELATIONSHIP OF WELLNESS EDUCATION AND HOLISTIC HEALTH

John W. Travis, M.D.

Wellness is a state of being, an attitude and an ongoing process, not a static state which we reach and never have to consider again. Most of us think of wellness as simply the absence of illness. But this is not accurate. There are degrees of wellness as there are degrees of illness.

Many people with no discernible physical illness feel bored, depressed, tense, anxious, or generally dissatisfied with their lives. Even without an identifiable clinical illness, there is a low degree of wellness. In fact, emotional states can lead to symptoms of physical disease by weakening the body's health and hence its resistance to illness. These emotional states may also lead some to self–abuse through smoking, drinking, or overeating. Such people are in the neutral point on the illness–wellness continuum (see figure 1).

The treatment model of both traditional or nontraditional ap-

This paper was subsequently published in slightly different form in Part IV of the *Wellness Workbook for Health Professionals,* © 1981, John W. Travis, M.D., reprinted here with permission. It is a special volume accompanying the Wellness Workbook by Regina Sara Ryan and John Travis (1981, Ten Speed Press, Berkeley, California). Both workbooks are available from Wellness Associates, 42 Miller Avenue, Mill Valley, CA 94941.

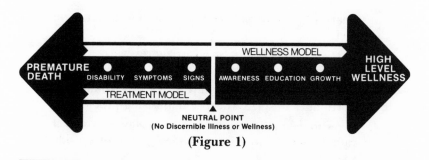

(Figure 1)

proaches is usually oriented towards curing the individual of the evidence of physical or mental disease; it does not necessarily help the individual to experience wellness.

The self–responsibility model does not provide for a relationship in which a patient expects a doctor to take care of him or her. Instead, people working with this model accept responsibility for their own well–being. Drawing from such fields of knowledge as physical fitness, nutrition, stress control, self–care and, for some, spiritual, transpersonal areas, individuals can learn to understand their basic emotional and physical needs and change their lifestyle in order to meet those needs.

These attitudinal and lifestyle changes take people beyond the neutral point. The treatment model cannot take them beyond this point because there are no definable negative conditions to treat. When a person is on the left side of the continuum, both models are useful in moving towards greater wellness. At this stage there is both a need for treatment and a need to learn the lessons the feedback from the disease can provide.

WELLNESS EDUCATION

Teaching people how to actively accept responsibility for their own state of well–being is what wellness education is about.

Two hundred years ago Karl Friedrich Guass said, "I have had my solutions for a long time, but I do not yet know how I am to arrive at them." The purpose of wellness education is to help people get involved in the process of arriving at their own solutions.

Objectives

The objectives of wellness education are designed specifically to help you:

1. Learn what your real needs are and how to get them met.

2. Act assertively, not passively or aggressively.

3. Perceive diseases or symptoms not as problems, but as feedback messages from your body, providing opportunities to solve a deeper underlying problem.

4. Grow toward assuming total responsibility for yourself rather than feeling like a helpless victim of outside sources.

5. Be the change you want to have happen rather than trying to change those around you.

6. Express yourself creatively.

7. Allow your vulnerabilities to surface, and be able to disclose yourself in safe situations, rather than creating tension within yourself by pretending you have no "weaknesses."

8. Cultivate a basic sense of well–being, which you can appreciate even in times of adversity.

9. Learn how to create and cultivate close relationships with others.

10. Engage in continual growth and transformation.

11. Choose to experience peace rather than conflict, guilt, or blame.

12. Respond to situations with love rather than conflict, guilt, or blame.

13. Accept the inherent paradoxes of the universe.

14. Trust that you already have everything you need available within you.

15. Experience yourself as a wonderful person.

THE WELLNESS RESOURCE CENTER

I founded the Wellness Resource Center in 1975 in Mill Valley, California, now known as Wellness Associates. Wellness Associates offers people resources to increase their own levels of wellness. A working principle is that wellness is enhanced when an individual assumes more responsibility for his or her own physical, mental, and emotional health and well–being. The task is to determine how an individual learns to assume greater responsibility. The following is a description of our response to this task.

The major resources we use are practitioners, programs, and publications. There is also a library of books and audiovisual materials and a resource file of wellness–related activities in the San Francisco Bay area.

The program can be divided into five areas, which include:

1. *The Wellness Evaluation.* This Wellness self–assessment is based on the Wellness Index, a series of 300 questions found in the Wellness Workbook and published separately. These questions focus on lifestyle, life view, and living habits, with emphasis on how they relate to health and well–being. You have a 3–hour conference with one of the practitioners. Included, too, is the taking of biofeedback and other physical measurements, and an exercise to assess your level of creativity.

2. *Being Aware of Your Body.* Biofeedback, massage, and other body–awareness techniques can help you let go of the "armor" which stress often creates in the body. Stress can be defined as the result of holding an opinion of yourself that is inconsistent with the way you really are.

3. *Taking Care of Your Body.* In an individualized process, you learn to consider your diet and needs and wants—from talking about specific attitudes which discourage proper self–care, to taking a tour of a whole foods store, to going outside and running with a practitioner.

4. *Taking Charge of Your Mind.* This involves one–to–one counseling for strengthening your ability to actively create your life circumstances rather than simply react to them. Zen–like question–and–answer techniques and "be here now" processes help attenuate self–defeating, stress producing thoughts and attitudes, mental habits, and automatic reactions to situations. Sessions can focus on improving specific areas of life, for example, relationships, money, sex, job, work, or can engage the more general areas of life goals and confidence in yourself and the future.

5. *Communicating Your Needs.* This takes place in private sessions as above or in a "Lifestyle Evolution Group" with a trained leader. The emphasis is on: learning skills for healthy and enjoyable living;

letting go of tension; communicating clearly; knowing more fully what emotions are being experienced at any given time and using those emotions to effectively solve problems; and structuring life so that basic human needs, especially self–nurturance, are met.

WELLNESS EDUCATION AND HOLISTIC HEALTH: NOT SYNONYMOUS

Our program of wellness education assumes that symptoms and illness represent only the iceberg tip of "dis–ease." We do not provide medical services or treatment. Instead we focus on ways in which each person can come to understand and change the underlying attitudes which may lead to disease.

People who come to us are called "clients," not "patients," to emphasize the importance of the commitment to self–responsibility.

Because of our alternative approach to health, many place it in the same category as holistic health–care practice. While supportive of the less "flaky" elements of holistic health, Wellness Associates is not a holistic health treatment center. We follow the self–responsibility model which can differ significantly from the treatment model.

Confusion may arise from similarities. Both the Wellness Associates and holistic health practitioners view the human body as a whole, a totally interrelated, interdependent organism. Both focus on the person, not the disease. Both promote the interrelationship and unity of body, mind, and spirit.

In contrast to traditional allopathic (attempting to alleviate symptoms) medical doctors, wellness and holistic practitioners do not, in most cases, treat clients with drugs or surgery.

However, while there is much greater emphasis in holistic health than in traditional medicine on people taking charge of their own health, its primary orientation is often still towards healing conditions of illness. In contrast, the primary orientation of wellness is on increasing conditions of wellness.

Usually, a holistic health practitioner specially trained in a certain discipline directs the treatment. In this sense, while the recipient of the treatment often learns much more about it than in traditional methods, there is usually a necessary dependence on the practitioner relationship by the person undergoing the healing process.

This relationship while perhaps not undesirable, may be limited in usefulness. When a person is sick, it is often appropriate to "borrow" energy from someone through a dependent relationship.

During the recovery period and especially afterwards, a person can prevent many future problems by understanding the meaning of the "advantages" it bore. These next steps are sometimes overlooked in the treatment model be it traditional or holistic.

In the beginning of any relationship with a wellness practitioner, there is a certain amount of dependence, and expectation of "being cured." This seems unavoidable. Rather than encouraging this stage, however, it is acknowledged and minimized, and the goal of fostering independence is reinforced.

OTHER RELATED MOVEMENTS

There are also several major alternative movements in the health–care field which I would like to distinguish from wellness education. Health promotion is in some ways a remodeling of old health–education principles which may sound great but haven't been effective. It often focuses on one issue such as physical exercise or diet or relaxation. This can be likened to a political rally where everyone is expected to fit in a mold and support the cause no matter what his or her own needs are.

Medical Self–Care is a movement attracting forward–thinking practitioners and students within the medical establishment. It aims to educate potential patients to take care of themselves intelligently. In some cases specific wellness methods are promoted, but, for many of its followers, the focus is only on what to do when something goes wrong, and how to participate more fully in the curative process.

While not specifically oriented towards physical health, humanistic psychology, the consciousness–expanding movement, and spiritual movements all recognize that health is a reflection of one's mental attitude. Many wellness concepts are similar to concepts originating in these disciplines. The latter, however, often tend to focus on elevating the leader, therapist, or guru to an authority role. I believe this weakens the message of self–responsibility.

A THREE-DIMENSIONAL MODEL RELATING HEALTH DISCIPLINES

To display the relationships between the disciplines associated with wellness and holistic health, I suggest a three dimensional model representing three continua between polar opposites: wellness–illness, holism–atomism, and the client–healer orientation.

The Model

Begin with the one–dimensional Illness/Wellness continuum (Figure 1), which we have already discussed. Add it to a second, vertical dimension showing holism in the upward direction and atomism (splitting things into the smallest recognizable components) in the downward direction (Figure 2).

This gives us a set of Cartesian coordinates. A discipline in the upper left quadrant would be illness–oriented and holistically approached. Similarly, a discipline located on the line between the lower two quadrants would be both illness and wellness oriented but atomistically approached.

A third dimension can be represented by a perspective drawing (Figure 3).

Figure 4 is an expansion of Figure 3 in which the more distant oval represents disciplines at the healer end of the continuum. The second oval represents the midpoint on the client–healer orientation continuum. The third represents the client–oriented portion of the third continuum or dimension. By stacking the three planes we can visualize a three–dimensional model. To simplify the model I use only three locations on each of the three continua (at either end or in the middle), recognizing that in practice there is much greater variability.

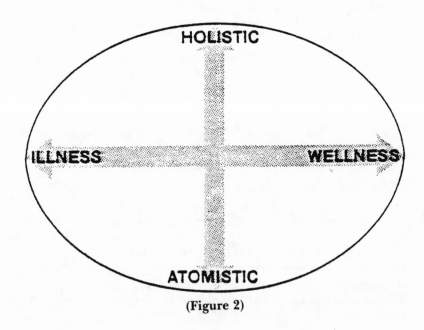

(Figure 2)

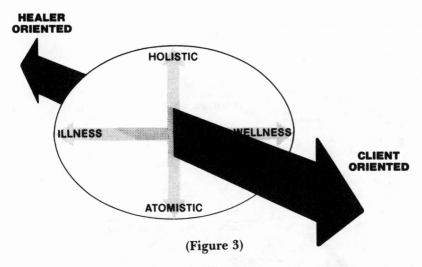

(Figure 3)

I have placed the major disciplines according to my personal experience with a limited number of their practitioners. The way individual practitioners choose to use these disciplines may locate them at different places on the continua.

While the model may imply a value judgment that wellness is better than illness, holism is better than atomism, and client–oriented is better than healer–oriented, my intention is to clarify how far removed wellness education is from traditional medicine. It also shows that wellness education and holistic health have considerable differences. I am espousing a relatively unrecognized area of health—wellness. To increase its impact, I present it in the foreground to contrast it with the better known disciplines.

Allopathic medicine is at the opposite end of each continuum from wellness. That does not mean allopathic medicine is bad, but that it entails certain risks and involves a need for treatment which is not within the domain of wellness education. For example, if I had acute appendicitis, it would be appropriate for me to choose a solution that (1) was illness–oriented, (2) was atomistically (surgically) oriented, and, (3) relied heavily on the healer (surgeon).

But during recovery I would be more interested in (1) the wellness approach: how I created and could prevent the occurrence of acute infection, (2) the holistic approach: how my diet and exercise relate to my illness and recovery, and, (3) how I can take greater responsibility for my self–healing through creative visualization and meditation. Each discipline has an important role to fill and each can complement the others.

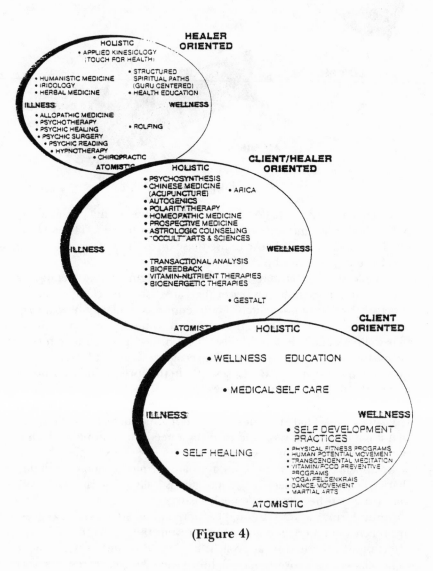

(Figure 4)

WHY DIFFERENT PRACTITIONERS FOR WELLNESS EDUCATION AND TREATMENT CARE?

A crude but useful analogy can be drawn from the automobile. Two separate systems exist, one for automobile repair (acute care/crisis intervention) and one for driver education (prevention/education). The automobile repair system is to the driver education system as the treatment model is to wellness education.

If I take my car in for a brake relining and front end realignment 5,000 miles after the last one, my mechanic, if there are good records to be examined, can be pretty sure I "ride" the brakes and drive over curbs or down rough country roads. Should he or she take the time to give me a driving lesson? It would seem more efficient for him or her to make a remark about the finding, ask a few questions, and then recommend a driver's training program. Possibly this mechanic could even share a building with driving counselors who could explain to me the relationship of my driving habits and my repair bills while I wait for my car to be fixed. Because there is little connection between the two professions, however, this rarely occurs. The mechanic may assume people are not really interested in improving their driving habits—or may have given up mentioning such observations. The need to keep to a schedule for working on cars may make it difficult, too, to get the message delivered.

It is theoretically possible for one person to practice disciplines on different ends of a continuum with the same client. However, I believe this to be extremely difficult in practice, especially for physicians. My belief is based on two factors—the financial cost–effectiveness, and the authority figure status of physicians in the eyes of most patients.

The typical physician's training is very costly and geared towards acquiring expertise of a highly specialized technical nature, much of which is related to treating the pathological functioning of the human anatomy. Even if he or she were trained to educate people in wellness—in having some knowledge of the role of nutrition, fitness, emotional, and psychological needs in relationship to health—these areas were probably not those which attracted him or her into medicine and may be of little interest. To provide wellness education takes considerable time with the client and a commitment to the process, requiring patience and nonattachment to the client becoming the way you (the educator) would like her or him to become. Given the technical and costly nature of medical training, I question the cost effectiveness of concentrating energies on performing roles other than those requiring a physician's more specialized skills.

There is also the problem of the authority figure role cast upon physicians by most patients. When physicians attempt to place the responsibility for health back in the patient's hands, they are often met with more resistance than practitioners seen as having less authority.

CONCLUSION

What the successful practice of wellness education requires is movement into a new paradigm, in which we see each individual as being as equally responsible and powerful as every other, recognizing the power of our feelings and actions, and our interdependence with each other. Such a movement involves a change in consciousness to one in which the basis of all actions is the realization that each person creates the realities he or she experiences. Within this paradigm each individual accepts him– or herself as fully responsible for his or her own being. There is no talk of changing others, or of knowing what's best for others. The environment is one of allowing others to be who and what they are, of being with them rather than doing to them.

I believe the ramifications of such a movement into a wellness paradigm go far beyond the manner in which we work with clients. It involves incorporating wellness into all aspects of our being, and how we relate to all other forms of life with which we share this planet. I believe that not only is the potential for such a movement within us, but that indeed the transformation is already underway.

Part VI

INTEGRAL MEDICINE
AND THE LIFE CYCLE

Though conventional medical care recognizes the need for different kinds of training for those who care for patients at different stages of the life cycle, it has done little to conceptualize or create the context for that care. It has tended, instead, to fit the challenges of each time of life into a pathological model. This may offer considerable hope to some, but it tends to narrow and distort the experience of others. In the last 50 years, for example, childbirth has been transformed into a medical emergency and old age a chronic and terminal disease. Those about to be born or to die—and those in between who fall ill— are often treated isolated from friends and families in impersonal institutions outside their communities.

The three chapters in this section help to reconceptualize the therapeutic approach to people in various stages of the life cycle, to restore them to their larger familial and social context. Richard Miles, in chapter 16, surveys some of the conditions which have prompted expectant parents, physicians, and midwives to create new environments for birth.

Richard B. Miles is assistant dean for the Graduate Program in Holistic Health Education at John F. Kennedy University in Orinda, California, and also lectures in the Health Science Department of San Jose State University. He is coauthor of *Freedom From Chronic Pain* (J.P. Tarcher, Los Angeles, 1979), and contributor to *The Holistic Health Handbook* (And/Or Press, Berkeley, 1978) and *The New Healers* (And/ Or Press, Berkeley, 1980).

In Chapter 16 Dennis Jaffe introduces readers to the ways in which recent developments in family therapy are helping clinicians to understand and treat physical illness in its familial context.

In Chapter 17 Evelyn Mandel and Jan Harlow describe an experiential program in which old and young persons work together to find the strength to overcome disabilities for which no medical treatment has yet been effective.

Evelyn Mandel founded the Institute for Creative Aging in 1975 to demonstrate that the elderly could be revitalized—their mental, spiritual, and physical health improved—through an eclectic program which tried new solutions to old problems. The premise of her program was that deterioration and disease do not necessarily accompany aging; the old fail only when growth and development are denied. Ms. Mandel is vice-president of the Center for Integral Medicine, a consultant with family gerontology associates and coauthor of *The Good Age Cookbook*, (Houghton–Mifflin, 1979) and *The Art of Aging* (Winston Press, 1980).

Jan Harlow is president of Harlow Associates, a communications company that produces advertising copy, marketing strategies, news stories, environmental–impact reports, financial proposals, brochures, and scientific reports. Ms. Harlow is a member of the Board of Directors of the Center for Integral Medicine, member of the Board of Directors of the Institute for Creative Aging, and coauthor of *The Good Age Cookbook*, (Houghton–Mifflin, 1979).

Chapter 15

THE RITUALS OF CHILDBIRTH

Richard B. Miles

Medical specialists in the last century have dramatically increased their technical competence but have often done so by sacrificing the "human side" of childbirth. In recent years, a tide of concern and dissatisfaction with this trend has been rising. Large numbers of parents and health–care professionals are now asking questions such as "What sorts of priorities attend the event of birth?"; "How can people best express their personal feelings about their own birthing experiences?"; "What are the effects of drugs, forceps, anesthesia, fear, and anxiety on the baby and its parents?"; "Does separation of the newborn from its parents hurt the baby and impair a critical bonding process?"; "Why are low–risk deliveries treated as medical emergencies?"

As one facet of change, more and more people are seeking alternative birthing procedures. Two alternatives, in particular, to the standard Western medical model of birthing have come to the fore in the last few years. Although there is certainly room for argument about terms, we shall call them "the holistic model," and the "integral model." In this paper I will speak as an advocate of the latter model.

THE TRADITIONAL HOSPITAL BIRTH

The Western medical model of birthing arose as a reasonable reaction to the dangers of infant and mother mortality and as a way of decreasing the risk and pain to the mother of unattended births. It is also the fruit of our increasing use of, and dependence on, technology. At its worst, it treats childbirth as "a surgical operation at the end of a 9–month disease." At its best it offers the possibility of a healthy, normal infant and mother in cases where previously damage and death might have occurred.

A brief caricature of traditional hospital birth may serve to illustrate its negative aspects. The prospective parents' flight to a distant hospital starts at an inopportune time. In the movies this is always a scene of high comedy. In real life, it can be anxiety–provoking and sometimes tragic.

Once they have arrived at the hospital, the situation is less critical but hardly comfortable or inviting for the parents–to–be. The mother is placed in a wheelchair and rushed off to be "prepped" in a suitably sterile atmosphere. The father is left at the admission desk to cope with countless forms that could have been filled out and filed weeks before. While fathers are now generally allowed to accompany their wives into the delivery room, when the two are reunited depends on the baby's timing and the father's speed of writing.

No matter how well–prepared for delivery the mother may be, the straps, immobility, masks, glaring lights, and physical jostlings and proddings may leave her feeling trapped and powerless in a strange and frightening situation. If he has caught up with her, the father may feel as confused, frightened, and helpless as she. The tension of the delivery room is high for adults; it may be even more stressful for the newborn.

The infant shrieks as it is passed, handled, and aspirated. Thrust into its mother's arms for a few moments, it is quickly taken away and whisked off to the nursery for its own admission procedures. Except for its brief time in its mother's arms, the infant is treated as an object without personal involvement in the event of its own birth, a non-conscious, nonexperiencing thing, who will not really begin to interact with the environment in significant "learning" ways for weeks or months.

The mother is sent back to her room to recover from her ordeal. If the father is still with her, he may in some small way comfort her for the vague feeling that she and the experience are incomplete. She has been treated as a disabled person undergoing a high–risk surgical procedure, someone incompetent to manage the birth of her child or to relate to her infant. She has been, simply, a person to be managed.

The father, also passive, has likewise been a nonparticipant, a nervous and potentially intrusive bother. The physician, by contrast, has been the "manager" of the event, protecting the mother from the risk and pain of birth. Death and disfigurement have been lurking in every shadow, and fear of them has been in control. The roles of parents and infant alike have been subordinated to the implied dangers and the need to be prepared to prevent death at all costs.

ALTERNATE BIRTH SCENARIOS

An ever–increasing number of "natural" home births are being undertaken by parents today. These constitute what I call the holistic model. Here, the mother tells the father when labor pains have begun. Close family and friends are notified and begin to gather in the house. The mother continues to move comfortably in familiar surroundings.

The physician and/or midwife arrives, evaluates the condition of the mother and the baby, and remains in attendance as a sympathetic and reassuring, but not overwhelming, presence.

The mother has learned breathing and relaxation techniques to help her deal with pain. A familiar environment and the quiet encouragement of known and trusted family, friends, and professionals reduce her anxiety about unexpected events and feelings. She feels comfortable, in control.

The new person is welcomed into a warm, friendly environment prepared for his or her entrance. The mother takes the infant to her, caresses it, croons to it, seeks its eyes which are open and attentive. Each person who is present has the opportunity to feel a sense of attachment to this new being, to experience the wonder of its birth. Relationships are established which may never be broken.

After a short time, most of those present retire to other parts of the home to quietly celebrate the event. The mother and father and perhaps a close friend or relative remain with the infant for quiet bonding and mutual support. Soon the mother and infant sleep.

Descriptive words and phrases for the Western model include: risk avoidance, fear, efficiency, centralized, impersonal, impermanent, managed, anxious, separated, alienating, and noisy. By contrast, home birth may be characterized by such words as: loving, caring, personal, shared, relaxed, quiet, and warm.

In the holistic model, the infant is considered to be a highly con-

scious, perceptive, "open" human being who is seeking immediate interaction with other members of the species and other events in the
birth environment. Mothers are felt to be "birthers" with a long tradition of natural experience, persons who seek fulfillment from an
experience of birth which is itself a natural process and an integral
and vitally important part of family life. The father is a participant
and supporter—a coach, assistant, and partner. The physician or
midwife is an educator and expeditor, an experienced observer looking
for potential danger, a wise and interested partner rather than a remote authority figure.

THE INTEGRAL BIRTH MODEL

Recently, a third model for birthing has been developed, one
which has been called the "integral model." Those who adopt this
model have concluded that it is not necessary to ignore or forego the
many valuable contributions medical science has made in decreasing
infant mortality and morbidity in order to enjoy a family–centered,
natural birth.

In the integral model when labor begins participating members
of the family, often including children considered mature enough to
share in the experience, gather at a specialized birthing center in or
near a back–up hospital. Motel or hotellike family–style accommo-
dations are ready and waiting in a facility shared by other birthing
families. Though the facility is within or near a completely equipped
hospital, the environment has familiar homelike qualities and is relaxed
and quiet. The event is seen as a family process and not, unless it is
unexpectedly necessary, as a medical emergency. The midwife or birth
coach, who has been teaching and counseling the family throughout
the pregnancy, arrives to be with the family throughout the process.
This person is here to advise the family and reduce anxieties about
unexpected events, and also to monitor the progress of the labor in
order that the physician can be called later on, when birth is imminent.

There are few surprises for the parents and little technology is
required. Parents and professionals are assumed to be competent to
monitor signs of distress, and since there are concerned people on
hand at all times, "remote" observance such as fetal monitoring is usually unnecessary. The event of birth is unrushed, and the mother and
others have time to welcome the new infant, establish contact, and to
begin the bonding process. Should some immediate attention be required for the infant, it will be quite apparent to the alert professionals.

Hospital facilities are immediately at hand and are called upon. Should the birth proceed normally, time is allowed for prolonged maternal–infant contact before the routines of checking, measurement, first bath, and so forth, take place. The baby is quickly returned to the mother and family, and the professionals retire, leaving the birthing center to parents, siblings, and friends. On the average, the family will remain together in the center for one to three days after the birth.

This third option, which combines many of the benefits of the caring, family–centered view of birth with modern medical expertise, is now used increasingly across the country. Mt. Zion and San Francisco General Hospitals in San Francisco, Good Samaritan in nearby San Jose, and Santa Monica Hospital in Southern California are examples. The creation of these centers heralds a new era of parental–professional cooperation based on mutual respect and understanding. This model recognizes the importance of welcoming the infant into a warm, supportive environment, of establishing the parent–infant bond, and of providing parents with a sense of personal involvement in this significant life event.

RESEARCH ON BIRTHING

A number of studies, although for the most part preliminary and unreplicated suggest that we have tried too hard to manage or control the potential hazards of birth and that in the process, we have produced problems of great consequence. According to this work, we may have already reached what Ivan Illich has called "paradoxical counterproductivity." Some of these studies suggest that the integral model may offer a more effective and safer as well as a more humane approach to childbirth.

The work of Dr. Robert Mendelsohn, of the University of Wisconsin Infant Development Center, reported by Dr. Lewis Mehl in 1976 seems to illustrate this counterproductivity. Mendelsohn and Mehl recorded the results of over 2000 matched births for which there were no advance indications of special risk. Half of these were home births, while the other half took place in maternity hospitals. Among the hospital births, there were 30 significant birth–related injuries. There were none in the home births. Fifty–two infants required resuscitation during their hospital births in comparison to 14 born at home. There were six diagnoses of neurological damage to the children born in the hospital and only one such diagnosis among those born at home. These statistics suggest that, except for a predicted high–risk birth, the home may be a safer physical environment for normal birth.

Mendelsohn and Mehl's study is a preliminary one open to methodological criticisms. Those that have been done on the adverse effects of routine hospital birth procedures on maternal infant bonding and infant development are more sophisticated.

Dr. William F. Windle reported a long–term experimental study utilizing some 500 rhesus monkeys to simulate current hospital birth practices.[2] He found that four factors contributed to an overwhelming increase in the incidence of asphyxia neonatorum in the infants: (1) the use of the supine position for the mother, which prevents gravitational blood flow from the placenta to the infant and decreases by 25 percent the infant's oxygen supply; (2) premature severance of the umbilical cord, a routine hospital procedure, despite textbook warnings; (3) use of anesthesic drugs for the mother; and (4) labor–stimulating drugs—all too often used without medical indication, simply to fit a birth to the delivery–room schedule.

Introduction of these factors gave rise to: (1) the need for infant resuscitation; (2) prolonged respiratory distress; (3) diminished capacity of the infant to relate to the mother as demonstrated by the infants' inability to suck, cling, etc.; (4) severe motor dysfunction in early infancy; and (5) irreparable abnormalities in brain formation. Dr. Windle concluded: "A great many human infants have to be resuscitated at birth. We assume their brains, too, have been damaged. . . . Perhaps it is time to reexamine current practices of childbirth with a view to avoiding conditions which give rise to asphyxia and brain damage."

Studies by Dr. Marshall Klaus and John Kennell at Case Western Reserve Medical School suggest a species–specific pattern ritual between the mother and infant in the first hour or so after birth.[3,4] During the period of the infant's "quiet alert" behavior immediately following a natural birth, the infant seeks the establishment of a bonding relationship with its parent. This process of bonding involves direct intense eye contact, extensive touching and holding, soothing and crooning sounds from the mother, and mutual smiling. These cues may be signals that the infant seeks to be recognized and assured that this new "space" of life is one in which he is welcomed. Mothers and babies left to their own devices will often naturally and completely engage in this bonding behavior. The Western medical model of childbirth often drugs the mother, separates her from her newborn, and eliminates the opportunity for this bonding to develop. According to Kennell, these early extra hours of contact could have a more decisive effect than many hours of health education and volumes of child–rearing advice.

Follow-up studies to Klaus and Kennell's maternal–infant–bonding studies have been conducted by Norma Ringler.[5] They reveal that infants who have more intimate contact with their mothers during the hours and days postpartum will achieve developmental milestones significantly earlier than those who are separated by standard hospital procedures. Ringler found that by age five, the IQ's, speech, and language comprehension of these children were significantly superior to those of the control group.

Infants born in a modern technological environment may be met with bright lights, sharp noises, acid in the eyes, premature severance of the umbilical cord (resulting in oxygen deprivation and the need for resusitation), masked faces, and cold surfaces. One may wonder whether this extraordinarily stressful situation establishes an attitude of defensiveness and mistrust which persists into later life.

In contrast to the standard technological delivery room, some hospitals are now providing Leboyer–type facilities in which these conditions are reversed.[6] In a recent study by Maria–Therese Guichard, the effects were assessed of 120 births of women from a middle—class Paris neighborhood who were randomly assigned to Leboyer type delivery rooms.[7] None had requested the process, but all had it thoroughly explained to them at the time their labor began. The children born by this process (three groups of 40 each; now ages one, two, and three) have been given standardized psychomotor examinations and observed by researchers. Parents have also been interviewed.

The childrens' developmental quotient of 106 on a scale of 129 was significantly higher than the average of 100 for the control group. In addition, observation of the children showed that they were exceptionally adroit and clever with both hands, that they began to talk at an earlier age, that they displayed less than the normal amount of difficulty in toilet training and self–feeding than the control group, and that they seemed to be protected from manifestations of colic and shortness of breath.

The parents, too, may have been affected by the process. Guichard noted that the fathers of these children seemed to take an exceptional interest in them. Though only the mothers were invited to follow–up interviews, 80 percent of the fathers came. This was not the case with parents who had used the Western medical model of birthing. Guichard concluded that the Leboyer method may not only improve psychomotor development in the infant, but that it may strengthen the attachment bond and affect the relationships of both parents to their children.

These and other studies suggest that the manner and conduct of birth has long–range implications for both parents and child, and that traditional hospital births that focus almost entirely on physical survival and the needs of the attending professionals may damage both the children and their relationships to their parents.

CONCLUSION

Perhaps in the future every family will have birthing options in their community and sufficient information available to them so that an informed choice may be made. Some may prefer traditional high technology and "painless" hospital births which may gradually be modified as new information of their ill effects becomes more widely known. Some may prefer "natural" home births. Others may prefer the model of the "integral" birthing center. It is to be hoped the result will be more relaxed, successful parents who will enjoy a deep inter-personal bonding connection with their newborns and newborns who, perceiving a friendly, welcoming world, will find themselves more ca-pable of dealing with their personal futures in constructive, creative ways.

REFERENCES

1. Mehl, L.E. Home birth versus hospital birth: Comparisons of outcomes of matched populations. Presented at the Annual Meeting of the American Public Health Association, Miami Beach, 1976.
2. Windle, W.F. Brain damage by asphixia. *Scientific American*, October 1969. pp. 76–84
3. Klaus, M., and Kennell, J. *Maternal infant bonding.* St. Louis: C.F. Mosby, 1976.
4. Kennell, J. Extra postpartum contacts strengthen mother's ties to baby? *Pediatric News*, 1972, 6,7.
5. Ringler, N.E. Mother's language to young children and the effects of early and extended contact on the speech and language comprehension at 5. Paper presented at the Annual Conference of the National Association for the Education of Young Children, Dallas, November 1975.
6. Leboyer, F. *Birth without violence.* New York: Alfred Knopf, 1975.
7. R. Trotter, Leboyer's babies, *Science News*, January 22, 1977.

Chapter 16

THE ROLE OF FAMILY THERAPY IN TREATING PHYSICAL ILLNESS

Dennis T. Jaffe, PH.D.

As a family therapist, I look at human problems—whether psychological or physical—within the context of a person's most intimate relationships. In a decade of work I have seen how the family has a central role in the creation, maintenance, and alleviation of every aspect of human difficulty.

To mention the importance of the family in creating psychological disorders such as schizophrenia, depression, phobias, and sexual dysfunction, or in creating physical illness, is not to neglect or negate the presence of psychological or biological factors lying within the individual sufferer. Rather, taking the family perspective acknowledges that the individual is also shaped and molded by environmental factors.

The family is the most central and potent external force not only in shaping the individual personality and its difficulties but also in the expression of physical illness. Therefore, family therapy supplements other approaches to physical illness and psychological difficulty by considering that the family environment, which might add to the problem, may also be a key factor in overcoming it.

Family therapy is a style of psychotherapy, taught in most psychiatry departments, in which the primary patient or treatment unit is not the individual but the whole family. The aim of the therapy process is to change the way the entire family works together. Changes in patterns of family interaction have a clear and observable effect on many individual symptoms of distress.

For the first years of my work in family therapy, I stayed within the psychiatric section of the hospital, working with families containing individuals who had serious psychological difficulty. Then in 1974 I began to wonder whether chronic physical illnesses, many of which were termed psychosomatic, might to some degree also be the result of family processes. If so, people with physical illness might respond to family therapy.

I knew, for example, that psychosomatic illnesses were remarkably resistant to medical treatment at the symptom level. Some people come to clinics repeatedly with vague and diffuse complaints, while others can be relieved of their acute symtoms but continue their stressful life styles, which set them up for future difficulty. The situation is similar in psychiatric clinics, where family therapy has proven helpful. Certain behavioral and emotional difficulties, which had been difficult to treat with either drugs or individual psychotherapy, were overcome when the whole family became part of treatment and the ways that family members interacted were explored.

In my experience there is a clear connection between physical illness and psychological or family distress. Initially, I began to talk to medical patients and to their family members sitting in the hospital waiting room about what was happening in the family before the illness, how they did things as a family, and how illness affected them. I found them eager to talk, and most felt that their relationships, family history, and conflicts were indeed important factors in the current illness. Yet few of those concerns were communicated to the physician, who was not attuned to such dimensions and did not consider altering family relationships as a goal or aspect of treatment.

My own role evolved from the conversations with patients' families. I saw myself as a partner with the physician, as one working with the family factors. Just as the physician's role was to alleviate symptoms by intervening at the individual's biological and physiological level, my role was to help the family change the parts of their lives that contributed to stress, hindered rehabilitation, or led to conflicts that were likely to become expressed as physical illness.

While every physician knows that emotional, environmental, and other stress factors are significant in creating illness, medical training does not currently offer the physician any tools for altering family conditions, other than caring concern and common sense. Any member of the medical team—a psychologist, nurse, social worker, aide, or technician—can be trained in a few months to offer rudimentary family therapy. For it to be effective, however, the physician must learn enough about family treatment to support and reinforce the work of other team members. It is my hope that the use of family therapy in treatment of physical illness will not simply be confined to the psychotherapist's office, but rather will become an integral part of comprehensive medical care, taking place within the medical clinic.

DYNAMICS OF FAMILY ILLNESS

There are two interconnected pathways by which an aspect of family functioning can become part of a causal network, the outcome of which is some type of physical illness. The first pathway is through the stabilization and repetition of a dysfunctional behavior pattern. A common example is the family where a child is given sweets as a reward or as part of family gatherings. By learning to eat certain foods to excess because of their connection with love, warmth, and good feelings from other family members, a child begins a treadmill of dysfunctional family behavior that is probably transferred, in turn, to the next generation.

Many common family behavior patterns that bring short-term pleasure have long-term consequences that are destructive to health. I have observed many times that when an ill individual tries to change bad habits, the well-meaning but undermining responses of other family members—who continue to offer sweets, for example—effectively destroy his attempts to change. That process suggests the importance of altering family patterns to gain compliance with health regimens in situations where only one family member has become ill.

The second pathway by which family relationships contribute to illness is through the intervening variable of chronic stress. There are detailed accounts of how psychological, family, and social events can activate the body's stress response, which in turn is related to many forms of somatic illness.[1,2] Chronic stress, due to our personality patterns, relationships, and life styles, has been related to all of the most common and destructive illnesses today. Such aspects of family relationships as conflict, continuing anxiety, uncertainty, change, dislocation, or crisis create a stress response in the physiological system of each family member. That response, if not reversed, can help create or aggravate an illness, or make it difficult for treatment to overcome illness.

Between family processes and physical illness lie many intervening variables, such as constitutional predispositions, weak organs and body systems, personality make-up, individual ways of handling stress, and beliefs and expectations, which make it unlikely that any clear pathway can be found between a specific family pattern and a specific disease. Instead of looking for simplistic cause-and-effect pathways, the family therapist must look at the uniqueness of each family and how the specific history and patterns of relationship and attachment may lead to different physical consequences in each family member.

There has been little research on the relationship between family interaction and physical illness. In a recent review article, Weakland notes that "family somatics" has been almost entirely neglected since a pioneering review article by Jackson more than a decade ago.[3] The results of most of the research have an unfortunate tendency to characterize family patterns as givens rather than as variables that can be changed. Yet family therapists have shown that even a relatively brief intervention (ten sessions) can alter longstanding family patterns.

My own work with more than 50 families in the Learning for Health program suggests that short-term family therapy can be a useful addition to the treatment process for many illnesses. In order to document its usefulness, review some of the literature, and suggest how individual families help create and complicate illness for their members, I will present accounts adapted from my work.

STRESSFUL LIFE EVENTS

A 30-year-old divorced woman with a young child has had three operations in the past year—for gallstones, for an ovarian cyst, and exploratory surgery—and was not recovering well from her last operation. She had recurrent pains, and was afraid of dying. Before this year she had no serious illness. She dated the onset of her troubles to her father's sudden death just two months before her first surgery. At the funeral she had a fight with her mother and younger sister and had not seen them since. She adored her father, whom she was much closer to than her mother, and she felt that her role in the family came about through her connection with him.

Between the first and second operation she broke off a long-term relationship with a man who was warm and loving to her, like her father. She was extremely upset and disoriented by her recent life changes, none of which had been addressed in her medical treatment. In talking to me, she began to explore her feelings about each of the changes in her family, and began to develop a new way of relating to her family. She was able to mourn her father's death, discover new ways to relate to the others in her family, and begin to think about having other deep relationshps.

In addition to the stress and change in her external life, she was under pressure because of the way in which she interpreted the stressful events. Her personal reactions to them included feelings that she was somehow responsible, that she ought to have died instead, and that she couldn't live without her father. As she explored these feelings and changed some of her intimate relationships, she began to heal.

FAMILY EVENTS AND ILLNESS

Astute physicians have always linked family events to illness. Parkes and others found that widowers were five times more likely than norms would suggest to die soon after their spouses, often of the same illness.[4] LeShan has reviewed scores of studies on personality, emotions, and family variables in relation to cancer, and he finds many studies supporting the association between cancer and loss of a person or object that is emotionally significant.[5,6] Thomas and Duszynski report on a prospective study of medical students that began more than 20 years ago. Their long-term data suggest that certain childhood family patterns can be linked with certain types of emotional and physical illness occurring many years later.[7]

The definitive research on the association between stressful life events and illness comes from the work of Holmes and Rahe and their associates. They developed a scaling procedure to rate the relative degree of adaptation required for the common life events of an individual. The Social Readjustment Rating Scale is a list of 42 common events; each event has a weight of severity ranging from 1 to 100. At the extreme end, 100, is death of a spouse; in the middle, at 50, is marriage; and at the low end are minor traffic fines, vacations, and holidays.

They found a series of studies that people, like the woman reported above, who have a number of serious life changes within a year—whether positive or negative—are at risk for serious illness. Their research suggests that any sort of adaptive change entails physiological stress, which may in turn lead to illness. Significantly, the majority of the important life changes on their scale are related to changes in family relationships.[8] In my work I have found that even the anticipation of life events or changes can be a precursor to illness.

SECONDARY GAIN

Nearly all of us, when we were children, occasionally exaggerated a pain to stay home from school and received an unusual outpouring of affection and care from a worried mother. That is an example of what is termed secondary gain—a positive consequence of an otherwise negative condition.

Every physician observes how disability, chronic pain, and illness can bring a family member benefits and can excuse him from some responsibilities. It is my observation that secondary gain is present in a majority of illnesses and thereby contributes, probably not at a conscious level, to some people's reluctance or inability to get well.

A striking example of how secondary gain may affect illness came from the family situation of a woman with cancer. Her husband was suddenly transferred to a new office in a different city, and she had to leave her home of 20 years. During the same period, her children had been leaving for college. After the move it took her a few lonely years to make a place for herself. Her husband worked long hours during that time to earn another promotion. Finally she felt at home.

Once again, however, her husband announced that he had to move. She developed breast cancer. As a result of her treatment, he was unable to move. She did not respond to chemotherapy. During family therapy, she was asked what would happen if she got better. "We would move, and I would have to find a whole new set of friends," she replied.

I do not know how much the couple's subsequent agreement to stay in their current home, and the husband's decision to spend more time vacationing and doing things with her, had to do with her current remission. After therapy, however, which involved airing her feelings about not being taken into account in decisions, she did better in medical treatment. The work of Simonton and Simonton offers many further examples of the association of secondary gain with poor response to cancer treatment.[9]

Another aspect of secondary gain comes when one family member's sickness seems to be a way to compel attention, affection, care, or simply time from the mate or parent. Illness is often a part of family life in ways similar to alcohol. The ill person, like the alcoholic, is presumed to be helpless and infantile because he or she is "ill," and consequently gets a great deal of attention.

One of the most difficult aspects of family therapy is unraveling the sources of secondary gain in a family with an ill member. Yet in many cases where an individual becomes ill for no clear physical reason, maintains chronic pain, does not respond to treatment, experiences symptomatic recurrences after treatment, or simply does not return to health despite the success of medical treatment, secondary gain provides the key.

There are not only secondary gains for the ill person but also potential gains for other family members. For example, a sick child may keep a couple from having to spend time together, or help a wife keep away from her husband. Or nursing may be the most comfortable way for one spouse to show affection, so that person would encourage his or her mate to be sick as often as possible.

The many permutations of secondary gain all relate to its primary quality: through illness a person is able to exert control over other family members or get what he wants, without having to own up to the fact that that is what he is doing. It is not conscious, because the common assumption is "I can't help being sick; it's not my fault." Haley explores the effects of such denial of responsibility on relationships, and he offers guidelines for the therapist to help families to short-circuit these self-destructive pathways of communication.[10]

I explore potential sources of secondary gain by asking questions of family members. First I observe that sometimes a person gains certain advantages from being sick, and then ask them to explore what they might be in their or their relative's case. Or I may suggest that they write a list of reasons why the patient became sick, and why he is remaining sick. Most people resist this approach at first, but with prodding are able to come up with reasons.

The suggestions made by some family members often lead other members to share the hidden feelings and reactions they have to illness, and to think of ways that they can be more honest in asking for what they need from each other. I have never found a family or an individual who could not identify secondary gains from illness. It is not that I feel it is wrong to receive secondary gain, but simply that most people can learn to receive the gain without the cost in terms of illness.

LETHAL DYADS

I have seen several examples of what I have named lethal dyads—couples who escalate each other's potentiality for illness by the structure of their relationship and the nature of their demands on each other. The emotional and personality patterns of each person seem to bring disaster to the other. It is not simply a specific personality or emotional make-up that brings on illness, but the personality that lives in an environment in which another person acts in a certain way. Unless the pattern of the relationship is changed, each member of such a dyad literally drives the other to chronic illness.

An example is a middle-aged couple, both of whom were seriously ill. The husband, an engineer, described himself as a workaholic. He had a serious coronary and had to work less. His wife was diagnosed as having cancer soon after. In family interviews, it turned out that the husband had always been the responsible one in the family, a role that his wife willingly agreed to. She grew increasingly helpless and dependent on his taking initiative and responsibility. His illness almost forced her to switch roles and take initiative. At that point she developed cancer, which in turn worried him and made him feel he had to be more responsible, to pay the bills, and to take care of her. He couldn't let down, but experienced new demands, responsibility, and worry.

Thus a lethal cycle was in motion. His illness seemingly resulted in part from his taking on too much and driving himself too hard. When he was forced to become dependent and reverse roles with his wife, she reacted by having a breakdown herself—in effect trying to get him back into his accustomed role. It was not a conscious process, but it was hard for me not to feel that their illnesses were connected with this interaction pattern. I helped them to do some things for themselves and to help each other. Each began to recover.

Hoebel studied coronary patients who continued to ignore risk factors like diet, exercise, smoking, and lack of relaxation and were uncooperative in their medical treatment. His assumption was that their wives could affect their behavior and help them to give up their dangerous activities. So he asked only the wives to participate in the program. In several sessions, he helped them see that, although their intentions were good, they may not have been meeting their husbands' medical needs. He helped them develop and put into effect strategies that encouraged their husbands to change. Without the husbands' cooperation, he was able to influence them to change simply by helping the wives change their behavior.

His conclusion was that health-threatening behavior in a family is due to interaction, and that family treatment can be successful even with the highly resistant or noncompliant patient. Hoebel suggests that noncompliance is a family problem, and is amenable to family treatment. He showed that lethal interaction in couples can be reversed. If spouses can lead each other to illness, they can also learn to help each other regain health. Hoebel had demonstrated a corollary of family therapy: since a family system is interconnected, a change in any one part or person, not necessarily the patient, can result in positive change in the patient.[11]

I have found that any treatment regimen can benefit from work with the whole family, by promoting compliance and dealing with problems that arise as a result of caring for the ill member. Strauss suggests that the reaction of the family is the crucial determinant of the extent of rehabilitation from chronic illness.[12] Also, as noted in the couple above, the illness of one family member creates stress and changes the family situation for the others, and may in turn lead them to illness. When one family member is seriously ill, all other family members are at risk to develop illness. That is why family-oriented physicians must be alert to the results of one family members's illness on the others.

THE CHILD AS A SCAPEGOAT

The most comprehensive application of family therapy to physical illness has been in the work of Minuchin and his colleagues with children with anorexia nervosa, abdominal pain, asthma, and diabetes. They observed certain family interaction patterns in those illnesses, created a theoretical model of how psychosomatic illness is created within families, and tested the model.

Of several factors Minuchin suggests as necessary for the development of severe psychosomatic illness in children, one is that the sick child plays an important role in the family's pattern of conflict avoidance and that role is an important source of reinforcement for his symptoms. The ill child is, in effect, a scapegoat whose illness takes up the family's concentration and focus, thereby allowing them to avoid some other conflict.[13]

The way that the ill child short-circuits a parental conflict is illustrated by a family with an asthmatic child. Whenever the mother was angry at the father, she would confide in her ten-year-old son, telling him that he was the "only one who understood her." The father was cold and seemingly uninvolved in the family. The parents had no sexual relations. The mother seemed to put all her energy into her son, taking care of him, and in a sense asking him to never leave her emotionally the way his father did. As the child felt the conflict and the responsibility of his role, he obeyed his mother by becoming weak, aggravating a hereditary predisposition, and developing asthma.

Ill children, whether as a consequence or a cause of their illness (probably a little of both), tend to be protected by parents, and develop few relationships with friends and achieve little independence from their family.

Minuchin's treatment strategy usually involves helping the child to become more independent from the family, and convincing the family to be less concerned, intrusive, and involved in the child's physical state. At this state of treatment, the conflict or distance between the parents becomes obvious, as the child moves toward his friends. The parents' conflict must be addressed in the final stage of therapy. The parental conflict is not often obvious until the central focus on the child's illness is changed.

Following Minuchin's strategy, I helped this family accomplish several tasks. First, I tried to cut the secondary gain for the son by encouraging the family to send him to school and to play with friends. I had the physician reassure the family that he was not seriously ill and could be active without medical risk. That eased their anxiety somewhat.

Second, I tried to get the father to do more with his son. It turned out that both were interested in athletics, but the father had avoided them because he felt the son was not strong enough or interested. That suggestion helped the boy make contact with his father. The boy's attacks became less severe.

Soon I began to see the parents separately, and they began to see that they had very little to say to each other and spent very little time together. They also began to face the fact that their lack of sexual contact was hurting their relationship. They entered couples therapy to work on these issues, and the son's asthma receded from being a focus of their attention.

THE FAMILY THERAPY PROGRAM

My program, Learning for Health, involves applying to the area of physical illness family therapy techniques that have already been successfully applied to psychological difficulty. So far it has involved short-term individual, family, and group therapy—five to 15- hour-long sessions—as part of a comprehensive medical treatment program for a chronic physical condition.

My referrals come in almost equal numbers from individuals, their families, and physicians. The clients are often people who have had negative or inconclusive encounters with medical treatment and who want to explore psychological and family contributions to their illness. Since most of the clients have not had previous experience with psychotherapy, I do not feel that they are any more predisposed to believe that family factors are important than ordinary medical patients. However, they seek my help at a time when other approaches have failed and are eager to cooperate, as are their physicians. I tell prospective clients that my work is experimental, based on a hypothesis that family and psychological factors are important in illness and healing. I ask them to join me in an inquiry into the role of such factors in their illness.

While the work progresses differently with each couple or family, I have found that there are certain common elements that make up the total approach. They do not occur in any particular order, but they illustrate the range of activities that together fall within family therapy.

Family history. I always take a family history that includes how the family has developed over the last two generations, focusing on major events. I ask about illnesses and how the family reacted to illness; changes, transitions, crises, and scandals; personalities; and recent stress. I usually interview the couple or family together, focusing on each person in turn. Often I ask each person to write his autobiography between the first two sessions, to reflect on past factors that might contribute to illness. I also use a questionnaire that helps the family focus on their past in relation to their present concerns. That process takes from two to four hours, and often helps the family to make important connections without prodding or interpreting on my part.

Exploration of meaning of the illness. Whatever its physiological nature, I assume that an illness has a certain function, role, and meaning in the family. In asking how the illness is treated by the family, what it does for the ill person, and how it affects the family, I explore various secondary gains and also look for deeper symbolic significance of the illness for family members. Often the illness repeats a pattern of a generation earlier, such as an expectation that the ill person would die of the same disease and at the same age as a relative.

I ask the patient and other family members two questions repeatedly: why are you ill right now, and why did you first become ill? I let them find as many reasons as they can. My intent is to open discussion within the family that counteracts the common medical assumption that a person has nothing to do with his own illness. I ask families to explore the illness with the assumption that perhaps something they are doing, or have done, relates to its onset and severity. I let the family determine the relevance of their answers for themselves.

Education. Since my approach demands the active participation of family members, I need to educate them in an unfamiliar perspective on illness. Therefore, I give them some articles written by me and by others on psychological and family factors in medicine and on the relation of stress factors to illness. Each person also receives a personal health workbook and journal to focus his self-inquiry into illness. I also conduct classes in stress release, through meditation, imagery, or autogenic training, which I encourage all members of the family to attend. In addition, I furnish information about health habits and the role of behavior in maintaining health.

This remedial health education is one of the most meaningful and important parts of any total health program, although education is not traditionally conceived as part of either medical or psychological therapy. A discussion of readings on health can often precipitate important family insights about changes, and also is an important way to lead the family members to see that they are important to maintaining their health.

Contract to change. I help each family look at aspects of their interaction that they want to change, and support them in experiments to accomplish that change. At each session outcomes are evaluated, and subsequent steps planned. The relationship of all aspects of family life to the current illness are explored. I also make contracts with individuals to carry out changes, and work with family members individually when necessary.

System change. Following other family therapists, I try to change not only specific factors that may lead to illness but also general aspects of the whole family as a system. I have found that certain qualities of family interaction correlate with emotional and physical health. Those qualities include flexibility in sensing and responding to new situations; openness to and active seeking of information from friends, relatives, agencies, and schools; ability to express feelings so that other family members can respond accurately; and autonomy from the family so that each member can pursue outside interests and involvements.

Support group. I find that change can be maintained only when the environment supports it. Thus it is difficult for one member of a family to lose weight when other family members joke about it or bring home sweets. Changes in a family life style that support health and help individuals overcome illness are often hard to maintain. Therefore, I find that support groups, modeled after such groups as

Alcoholics Anonymous or Weight Watchers, can be important in maintaining changes once they have been made. As a final step in therapy I like to see one or more family members participate in a support group or follow-up treatment. Health is not a one-time achievement; it must be actively maintained.

My clinical experience indicates to me that family relationships, behavior patterns, and the way that people respond to stressful life events are important causal factors in illness and health. As yet there are only rough theories and a few scattered clinical observations that move beyond the basic assumption that family dynamics are important to health. More research is needed to show the physician, therapist, or member of the health team that it is important to include family therapy in the treatment program. Through family therapy it is possible to affect family relationships and stress factors in a positive direction, toward greater health.

References

1. Pelletier, K.R. *Mind as healer, mind as slayer.* New York: Delacorte, 1977.
2. Jaffe, D.T. *Healing from within.* New York: Bantam, 1982.
3. Weakland, J.H. Family somatics: a neglected edge. *Family Process,* Vol. 16, March 1977, pp. 263–272.
4. Parkes, C.M., Banjamin, B. & Fitzgerald, R.G. Broken heart: a statistical study of increased mortality among widowers. *British Medical Journal.* Vol. I, March 22, 1969, pp. 740–743.
5. LeShan, L. Psychological states as factors in the development of malignant disease: a critical review. *Journal of the National Cancer Institute.* Vol. 22, January 1959, pp. I–18.
6. LeShan, L. An emotional life-history pattern associated with neoplastic disease. *Annals of the New York Academy of Sciences.* Vol. 125, January 21, 1966, pp. 780–793.
7. Thomas, D.B. & Duszynski, K.R. *Closeness to parents and the family constellation in a prospective study of five disease states: suicide, mental illness, malignant tumor, hypertension, and coronary heart disease.* Vol. 134, May 1974, pp. 251–270.
8. Holmes, T.H. & Masuda, M. Life change and illness susceptibility. In B.S. Dohrenwend & D.P. Dohrenwend (Eds.), *Stressful life events.* New York, John Wiley & Sons, 1974, pp. 45–72.
9. Simonton, O.C. & Simonton, S.S. Belief systems and management of the emotional aspects of malignancy. *Journal of Transpersonal Psychology.* Vol. 7, January 1973, pp. 29–47.

10. Haley, J. *Strategies of psychotherapy.* New York: Grune & Stratton, 1963.
11. Hoebel, F.C. Coronary artery disease and family interaction: a study of risk factor modification. In P. Watzlawick & J.H. Weakland (Eds.), *The interactional view.* New York: Norton, 1977, pp. 363–375.
12. Strauss, A.A. *Chronic illness and the quality of life.* St. Louis: Mosby, 1975.
13. Minuchin, S. et al. A conceptual model of psychosomatic illness in children. *Archives of general psychiatry,* Vol. 32, August 1975, pp. 1031–1038.

Chapter 17

CHANGING THE FOCUS
FROM DYING TO LIVING:

The Institute for Creative Aging

Evelyn Mandel
Jan Harlow

THE AGING PERSON

We are all aging. For most this means resisting, as best one can, the slow but inexorable loss of well–being, status, power, vitality, attractiveness, and even responsibility for the conduct of one's very own life. Vast amounts of money and effort are spent trying to deny or stave off the process of, and depth of fear surrounding the prospect of aging.

It is a problem of our time and culture that we reject participation by the senior population, devaluing their potential contributions and denying them meaningful activity. Statistics on depression, dependency, the effects of isolation, and the increase in psychiatric problems among the aged leave little doubt that present solutions to the problems of the elderly are, at best, merely ineffective and, at worst, devastating to the well–being and self–esteem of older persons.[1–12]

Since insufficient medical and psychotherapeutic services are available even for the aged who have been diagnosed as requiring them, the great majority of seniors are left to cope with life stresses on their own. The result has been unnecessary pain and discomfort, dependence on drugs, depression, loss of self–esteem, general anxiety, fear of the future, and passivity. Yet is has been shown that with proper treatment many of the debilities of the aged can be reversed or ameliorated.

In the past few years a number of innovative programs for the aged have begun[13] using self–help group concepts. They are based on the assumption that the aged have a far greater capacity for pleasure, productive involvement, physical health and vitality, creative pursuits, and for helping each other than has been commonly assumed. They treat chronic physical disability and teach methods of prevention that allow each person to maximize his or her capacity for living fully.

The programs are inexpensive, and involve group learning rather than individual consultation. They employ methods of human growth and psychotherapy which have been used with younger people at growth centers and in psychotherapy programs. They assume that the key to health lies in a daily regimen of activity and productive involvement rather than in conventional treatment of individual symptoms of decline. As other holistic programs, these focus on the individual as a whole, learning, growing, changing person.

The first of these projects was the SAGE Program, created in San Francisco by Gay Gaer Luce. It began by word–of–mouth, meeting wherever available space could be found, and employed methods that were taught to volunteer trainers and teachers and a small staff. The program's basic concepts and philosophy have since been used in a variety of other settings. One such project, the Institute of Creative Aging, described in this paper, exemplifies this new approach to improving the quality of life for the aged. The primary objective of the Institute is to show that an innovative, holistic program can revitalize elderly people and improve both their mental and physical health. We also hope to demonstrate that the project's approach and techniques can be transmitted to other lay teachers and geriatric professionals in a training internship program. Future plans include adapting the project's approach to community facilities which serve both ambulatory and nonambulatory participants, in senior centers, community–service groups, and board–and–care facilities.

THE INSTITUTE OF CREATIVE AGING PROGRAM

The core program of the Institute has 20 members, a staff of five instructors, a director, a counselor, and a medical consultant, functioning under the guidance of a Board of Directors. The group meets once a week for three hours and the staff meets one day a month to review the program's effectiveness and to consider possible modifications.

The staff was carefully selected for skills, sensitivity to people, and interest in and understanding of the aging process and, in particular, of their own aging.

The staff meets regularly with a psychotherapist to discuss and gain insight into how they are managing their own aging. The program assists elderly people in utilizing their physical, emotional, and spiritual potential, and in assimilating new attitudes that promote increased confidence in their ability to engage in everyday activities. By gradual extension of these activities, the self–renewing process is accelerated.

The program has selected a group of teachings and exercises culled from Western therapeutic methods and Eastern philosophies and synthesized them into a balanced group participation format. The basic program is comprised of meditation, group discussion, acupressure, Hatha Yoga, Tai Chi Chuan, and Feldenkrais methods. It responds directly to those problems most frequently encountered in the elderly, is noncompetitive, requires no special equipment, is not strenuous, and can readily be practiced alone at home. In addition, the Institute for Creative Aging offers support and guidance in total nutrition—the proper nourishment of the mind, body, and spirit.

Each meeting begins with a meditation, a time when participants can bring themselves to a quiet place and become aware of the important issues in their lives. Following the meditation, members share their thoughts and concerns. In the early stages of group formation, the conversation deals with relatively commonplace issues of daily living. Later attention becomes focused on such important aspects of aging as adjusting to a life which lacks the money, mobility, influence, and productivity that was once available. Later yet, the group becomes more profoundly involved with death and with feelings about their own dying and the death of important peers.

After the sharing time, the group is led in a period of physical activity combining yoga, Feldenkrais,and Tai Chi Chuan. Later instruction in acupressure—a technique that has proved effective in relieving many common physical complaints—is offered. The remaining time is used to present didactic material. Because the group is concerned with health maintenance and the prevention of illness, nutrition is a subject of intense interest.

Members are continually sharing recipes which are nutritionally sound, economical, and practical to prepare in small quantities.[14]

Members of the group pay serious attention to their bodies and, with diligent practice of the techniques taught in the program, have been able to report reduction in drug use, decreased insomnia, greater energy, fewer visits to the physician, weight loss, cardiovascular improvement, and a marked upswing of morale.

The Institute's program includes the following modalities:

Acupressure, the application of finger pressure to acupuncture points, has been used for centuries to deal with the problems associated with aging. It is employed as a self–help tool to alleviate symptoms such as anxiety, fatigue, muscle stiffness and spasm, poor circulation, poor digestion and elimination, hypertension, headaches, and insomnia.

Art Therapy explores creativity and self–expression through art.

Biofeedback Training is a technique which allows the individual to monitor and gain control over certain autonomic functions by receiving instantaneous feedback from devices which measure brain activity, heart rate, circulatory function, and muscle tension. It is useful for alleviating insomnia, anxiety, high blood pressure, headaches, and other symptoms prevalent among the elderly. It is a technique which places the power for change in the hands of the individual and greatly expands the possibilities for self–control.

Feldenkrais Exercises focus on variations of traditional movement in a gentle, almost effortless manner. They are especially suited to the older person who has become restricted by reduced habitual movement patterns. These exercises utilize countless variations of simple movements that encourage participants to let go of old habits and to accept alternatives that increase the range of movement. These exercises concentrate on means rather than ends and help participants to sense difficulties and explore possibilities for self–correction. Improved self–awareness and self–image are the results of demonstrations of how the older persons can reverse habits of stiffness and limitation.

Yoga training emphasizes postures that affect body alignment, balance, circulation, and breathing, improving posture, circulation, flexibility, and breath capacity. Energy increases and mental processes clear presumably with systematic relaxation and normalization of the sympathetic and parasympathetic nervous systems.

Meditation is a mental exercise which yields positive cumulative effects for the meditator. As a physical process, it is relaxing. As a physiological process, it fosters improvement in an individual's health. As an overall system, it satisfies a need for tranquility previously met by drugs.

Meditation dissolves an individual's inner deposits of stress and brings strength and energy to the surface. Participants, then relaxed and confident enough to increase their own awareness of the obstacles around them, gain in their ability to deal with them.

Sense of community, the feeling of love and companionship which pervades the group gives members a new outlook on who they are and what they can do to render their own lives more meaningful. This promotes a sense of belonging that may have become undermined.

Nutrition is emphasized in lectures. The focus is on proper nourishment for the aged.

Tai Chi Chuan, which is practiced widely by the aged in China, improves the individual's sense of balance and control. It teaches one how to relax every muscle not in use, to gain flexibility of the spine and joints, and to sharpen concentration. It helps restore balance, rhythm, and eye/hand coordination.

TEACHER TRAINING

Once the original core–group members have developed a sense of renewed energy, these individuals may then enter into a second stage—the apprenticeship program. In this aspect of the program, these newly functioning leaders are taught in greater detail the modalities that were employed in their own revitalization. Following this apprentice training, these individuals have the opportunity to bring the Creative Aging program to their peers, to become once again employable, integrated members of society.

This transformation is often astonishing. Four of the original core–group members began apprenticeship training, each specializing in the mastery of one modality. When they had first joined the Creative Aging program, they had all exhibited symptoms of depression and ill health. After six months, each of them was teaching the program's techniques to peers and each was enjoying the benefits of marked psychological and physical improvement. One core member was suffering from diabetes and a heart condition which had required frequent hospitalization in an intensive–care unit. She was taking 18 different medications daily when she first joined the Creative Aging program. Currently she is taking only one medication, is teaching in the program, feels wonderful and is very proud to say, "I did it." In addition to training members the Institute has an internship program open to qualified persons interested in learning to teach Creative Aging techniques. The program is designed to train interns in these methods and to build warm, confident relationships, first between trainer and intern, and then between the intern and the elderly people he or she will work with during the learning period.

Interns may be students (graduate or undergraduate students in psychology, psychiatric social work, public health, or premed fields), professionals or paraprofessionals (physicians, dentists, psychologists, nurses, physical or recreational therapists, social workers, or paraprofessionals at a geriatric facility), or other qualified persons presently working with the elderly. The Institute is able to train four to eight interns every six months.

Interns receive instruction and supervision from our staff in groups that meet for several hours each day. Individual assistance with specific problems is also available.

A crucial part of the internship training is attendance and apprenticeship in one of the ongoing core groups of elderly clients. Three interns are assigned to each group of 12 to 15 elderly clients. For 6 months these interns work with members of the group, participating in the learning processes and assisting in the leadership of group sessions. During this period there is ample time for each intern to gain necessary experience with a variety of skills and methods for working with the elderly.

EVALUATION

At the beginning of each program, the Institute's medical consultant and staff measure each member's blood pressure. They conduct follow–up checks at the middle and end of each 6–month program. To date, the data suggest that the Creative Aging techniques can play a significant role in reducing hypertension and keeping blood pressure down.

Dialogues with individual members have been the most fruitful source of information about the program's effectiveness. The primary difficulty in isolating techniques and describing results stems from the premise of the integrated approach and the interrelationship of effects from all the modalities employed. However, some measure of the effectiveness of different techniques may be inferred from limited but suggestive evidence.

Tai Chi Chuan was used at home by only 30 percent of the core group, but all of these reported significant improvement of balance, rhythm, and eye/hand coordination.

Acupressure is used by nearly every member at home, 75 percent reporting relief of such problems as headache, muscle tension, fatigue, insomnia, poor circulation, constipation, diarrhea, sinus congestion, edema, and hearing loss. Stimulation of "energizing" points seems to improve members' general outlook on day–to–day living and to enhance their ability to fulfill personal goals.

Yoga improves posture, circulation, flexibility, balance, and breathing capacity according to the subjective reports of nearly every participant. It appears to be especially helpful to those members who had been afflicted with low back pain and chronic muscular tension. In addition, it contributes to an increase in energy, alertness, and cleared mental processes, perhaps by systematic relaxation and normalization of the sympathetic and parasympathetic nervous systems. Virtually every member reported improvement of mood as a result of using the yoga breathing techniques.

Feldenkrais techniques have enjoyed the greatest impact of all in improving self–awareness and self–image. They seem to demonstrate concretely to participants that old habits of stiffness and limitation can indeed be reversed. Discovering that deterioration and immobilization are neither inevitable nor irreversible seems to have produced a boost in self–esteem and confidence for nearly every member.

Meditation has been used with positive results by nearly 95 percent of the group. Most often meditators are pleased with their ability to stop the "mental chatter" which had prevented them from seeing clearly the issues relevant to their personal growth and well–being.

Lectures and studies of nutrition bring rapid and direct improvement. Almost one–half of the group felt better when they followed diets geared to the older person.

Biofeedback has only recently been added to the program so that its results are not yet available.

Personal and spiritual growth, experienced by every member to a varying degree, defies evaluation in all but the broadest subjective terms. By removing physical and mental obstacles to well–being, the program helps participants to make more creative use of their retirement years. As they abandon the myths of uselessness and incompetence which have constrained them, members are able to transform their lives and reclaim pleasure, accomplishment, fulfillment, and continued growth.

CONCLUSION

The demonstration that Creative Aging techniques have utility for revitalizing the elderly has important implications for existing programs for the aged. Indeed, in some cases a total revamping of the current approach to treating the elderly may be required. If these methods, which need to be systematically studied, can reduce or eliminate pharmacological treatment of psychosomatic symptoms (anxiety, depression, headaches, insominia, gastrointestinal problems, muscle aches, and the like), the aged will be significantly benefited. If they can help prevent further mental deterioration, many aged may be spared depression, dependence, and institutionalization.

REFERENCES

1. Brodz, SJ. Evolving health delivery systems and older people. *American Journal of Public Health,* March 1974, pp. 245–248.
2. Eisdorfer, C., & Lawton, M.P. (Eds.) *Psychology of adult development and aging.* The American Psychological Association, Washington, D.C., 1973.
3. Keith, P.M. Evaluation of services for the aged by professionals and elderly. *Social Service Review,* June 1975, pp. 271–278.
4. Prakash, C.S. Studies on aging and the aged in america. A selected research bibliography, CPL, *Exchange Bibliography, No. 714, December 1974.*
5. *Social and economic characteristics of the older population,* 1974, Bureau of the Census, U.S. Department of Commerce, Special Studies Series. No. 57. November 1975.
6. *The Nation and Its Older People.* U.S. Department of Health, Education and Welfare, Special Staff on Aging. Washington, D.C.: U.S. Government Printing Office. 1961.
7. Butler, R.N. Age–ism: Another form of bigotry. *The Gerontologist, 1969, 9,* 243–46.
8. Butler, R.N. The burnt out and the bored. *The Washington Monthly,* 1969, *1,* 58–60.
9. Butler, R.N. *Why survive? Being old in America.* New York: Harper and Row, 1975.
10. de Beauvior, S. *The Coming of Age.* New York: Putnam, 1972.
11. Looking forward to what? The life review, legacy and expressive identity versus change. *American Behavioral Scientist,* 1970, *14,* 121–28.
12. *Old age: The last segregation.* Ralph Nader's Study Group on Nursing Homes. New York: Grossman, 1971.
13. Karnes, L. Alternatives to institutionalization for the aged. CPL, *Exchange Bibliography.* No. 877. September 1975.
14. Mandel, E., & Harlow J. *The creative aging cookbook,* New York: Houghton–Mifflin, 1979.

Part VII

NEW DIRECTIONS
IN HEALTH CARE

Integral practitioners try to unite the functions of physician, clergyman and psychotherapist, to work with patients as members of family and social groups, to create a context in which people's ability to help themselves is maximized. Though some of the work described in this volume has proceeded within the bounds of the health–care establishment, much has taken place outside it. In the future, as these concepts become more acceptable, the boundaries between integral – or holistic or behavioral or humanistic –medicine and conventional health, and mental health care will blur. This will present integral practitioners with the opportunity to help change the larger health–care system; it will also expose them to the danger of co-optation.

In this concluding section, psychiatrist James Gordon and attorney Rick Carlson discuss some of the new directions that health care and mental health care may take. Dr. Gordon has worked with community groups–runaway houses, hotlines, crisis centers, shelters for battered women, holistic health centers–which in recent years have been able to offer comprehensive services without sacrificing innovative and responsive care. His paper suggests that these alternative services may offer cost–effective models for all health and mental health care. Mr. Carlson, a theoretician and organizer, calls our attention to previous struggles for health–care hegemony. He warns that integral medicine may, as it becomes absorbed into the mainstream, lose much of what is valuable and unique to it. Both Gordon and Carlson believe that a new, more holistic approach to health and mental health care must continue to evolve outside as well as within the mainstream of American medicine.

Rick Carlson, J.D. is President of the Health Resources Group, a firm that consults with public agencies and private industry on issues of health policy and health promotion. Mr. Carlson, who was formerly Chairman of Governor Jerry Brown's Council on Wellness and Fitness is the author of *The End of Medicine* (Wiley-Interscience, 1974) and coauthor of *Future Directions in Health Care* (Ballinger, 1978).

Chapter 18

ALTERNATIVES IN MENTAL HEALTH

James S. Gordon, M.D.

THE PROBLEM

Recent estimates suggest that as many as two out of ten Americans may be in "serious need" of mental health services.[1] Each year almost 1 percent of our population is admitted to mental hospitals. And each year we consume several billion doses of Valium and Librium. Millions of people are addicted—to barbiturates, heroin, methadone, and alcohol. Psychosomatic disease is endemic. We are a people sorely troubled, desperately looking for some answer to our problems or at least some relief from them.

Too often we forget that these problems have roots in the particular conditions of our society, and that any attempts to achieve mental health must be inseparable from efforts to create a just, decent, and personally fulfilling society. We know that poverty predisposes people to psychosis and hospitalization; that fragmenting community structures and confused family relations promote depression, alcoholism, and schizophrenia; that pressured and alienating working conditions precipitate psychosomatic illness and drug use; that lack of employment opportunities and isolation and institutionalization depress older people. Yet we ignore this and focus our therapeutic attentions and our economic resources on individual sufferers. We call them "mentally ill," and all too often—as if their problems were simply analogous to a physical illness—treat them with drugs and electroshock therapy. When they do not get "better" we lock them up in mental hospitals.

During the last several decades the mental health establishment has adopted two major approaches to the American people's problems in living: biomedical research and the establishment of community mental health centers. Neither has lived up to the enthusiasm with which it was heralded. Both have been flawed by the pervasive and narrowing influence of a medical model of mental illness.

Biomedical researchers, ignoring the total ecological context—whole people in families and communities, work places, and cities—have searched for the specific anatomic locations, the physiological and biochemical causes of schizophrenia, manic–depressive psychosis, depression, and anxiety. Similarly, they have experimented with medical and surgical cures—the right drug or the right operation, the right place in the brain to stimulate or depress—just as they might with treatments for diabetes or cancer of the lung.

The most dramatic product of early biomedical research was the development of the phenothiazine group of tranquilizers of which Thorazine is the best known. Their history and their limitations are instructive. When phenothiazines were introduced in 1954 they were heralded as the "cure" for schizophrenia, the salvation of State hospital patients. An immediate exodus from State and county hospitals was followed over the years by a leveling–off process. Twenty–two years later the percentage of the overall population in mental hospitals has decreased somewhat, as has the average length of stay, but the overall numbers of patients admitted has remained about the same.

Some of those who have been "maintained" on phenothiazines—or the other still more potent drugs that were soon developed—seemed to function well outside the hospital. But many of them have come to feel as constricted, as robbed of their full potential, by the stupefying and numbing effects of the chemicals as they had been by the hospital walls. They felt as embarrassed and degraded by their dependency on powerful drugs and authoritarian doctors as they had by their reliance on prisonlike institutions. And many of those who felt satisfied with the emotional level on which their medication kept them have found themselves experiencing severe physical side effects—impotence, extreme sensitivity to sunlight, chronic skin rashes, easy tiring, obesity, and the chronic, often irreversible debilitating neurological disorder, tardive dyskinesia.

The passage of the Community Mental Health Centers Act in 1963 was an even more important milestone. Hailed as a "bold new approach" by John F. Kennedy, it signaled a modification of the medical model, a growing sensitivity to the effects of poverty and social stress on the creation of mental illness; an increasing awareness of the possibilities of helping people to change by working with them, their families, and their communities to change their social situation. Community mental health centers were designed to help prevent institutionalization; to bring low cost, readily available mental health services, including individual and group psychotherapy, to large numbers of people; and to make—through consultation and education—changes in families, schools, and communities which would forestall the development of mental illness in their members.

In fact, the community mental health centers have never resolved the contradiction between a social and a medical definition of mental illness. Their legislative mandate depends on their responsiveness to community needs, on their capacity for helping people not to become chronic mental patients, and, ultimately, on their ability to change those conditions which make people mentally ill. But the political power, social prestige, professional status, and high incomes of their leaders come from their roles as doctors and mental health professionals. Too many community mental health centers simply perpetuate the medical model and in so doing provide inappropriate services.

In outpatient clinics that are little more than an aggregation of private therapists' offices, they may insist that people fit into one or another diagnostic category and predetermined therapeutic experience. Instead of providing the services—economic and educational, vocational, and counseling—that are necessary to help seriously disturbed people live successfully at home and in their community, they tend to obliterate anxiety about these problems with maintenance doses of antidepressants and phenothiazines. The consultation and education that they provide is often directed at strengthening the skills of other professionals—teachers, guidance counselors, etc.—rather than, say, changing the classroom conditions which frustrate students, teachers, and guidance counselors alike. Rarely do they provide services to people who, though needy, are unwilling to define and stigmatize themselves as mentally ill. Even more rarely do staff members spend substantial amounts of time in the community they are supposed to serve.

All during my medical and psychiatric training, I was deeply troubled by the institutional condescension and coercion with which the medical model was compounded—enforced medication, electroshock treatment, locked doors, and seclusion rooms—and by the narrowness to which it urged its adherents.

Doing psychotherapy with poor people in a community mental–health center, I became increasingly sensitive to the wrongheadedness of an ideology which emphasized talking about intrapsychic difficulties and largely ignored the day–to–day realities which confronted people when, after an hour, they left my office. I discovered how much faster some of the most troubled people would lose their psychotic symptoms if I devoted more of my energy to understanding the concrete and oppressive realities of their lives—and then helped them deal with those realities.

Driving one man to a welfare office; waiting with him; helping him prod its sluggish and indifferent bureaucracy into giving him emergency payments let him know more graphically than any words that I really did care about him. Afterwards he spoke much more easily of his personal problems.

Visiting a "paranoid" teenager in her home, I discovered that her parents were constantly invading and intruding—on her room, her mail, her bureau drawers, her phone calls, even the pockets of her blue jeans. I obviously had to take her seriously when she told me that "they're as crazy as I am." She couldn't possibly become less "paranoid" until they changed.

Working with a Crisis Intervention Team in the psychiatric emergency room of a municipal hospital I discovered that the vast majority of those who would have otherwise been admitted could be helped to stay at home. With the intensive involvement of the crisis team (a psychologist, a nurse, and three paraprofessionals) a family could pull together to help one of its members during a psychotic episode or suicidal depression. While they assisted family members in dealing with external problems (welfare, job, housing, food) the team used the crisis as a lever to help them understand the particular dynamics which had precipitated it. Often, in a few weeks, without hospitalizing anyone, they were able to help a family resolve a situation which had seemed intolerable.

During the time that I was in charge of a hospital ward I discovered how much better off psychotic patients—and staff—could be if they were simply treated with the respect due other human beings. In the context of a community in which they were given power over their own lives, in which they took part in making rules and in working out cooperative living arrangements, a group of so–called mental patients simply stopped being so disturbed. Given trust, or at least the possibility of it, by a staff that refused to disqualify their speech and behavior as symptomatology, the patients were often able to trust and get help from staff members; free to come and go, they tended to stay and try to work out their problems; allowed to regulate their own medication they tended to use it occasionally, only when necessary and avoided becoming dependent on it. "Everywhere else" one "chronic schizophrenic" young man told me, "I'm crazy; here I'm sane."

Still I concluded that the reforms that could be made within the context of traditional mental–health settings would be severely limited by the structure of those settings and by the ideology of mental illness to which the professionals who dominate them subscribe. When I entered the U.S. Public Health Service, I decided to look for places in which troubled people could be helped—and could help themselves—without so many constraints.

ALTERNATIVE SERVICES

Twelve years ago I began to work—as a consultant, researcher, and colleague—with alternative human services. I wanted to see if the ideology of professionalism really did make it more difficult to meet the needs of some troubled people; if changing the setting in which help was given and the set of those who were giving it made a substantial difference in the people who received it; if some of the culturally alien but side–effect–free techniques they were using with their clients—meditation, massage, acupressure—might contribute to promoting their well–being; and if the skills I had developed in my psychiatric training could be effectively shared with and enlarged by groups of dedicated nonprofessionals. I am still working with alternative services. I surely do not think they are the total answer to people's problems in living, but they are surely dealing with them in a way that is respectful, open–minded and effective.

Alternative services are approximately fifteen years old. Most of the early ones were founded by indigenous helpers, in direct response to the physical and emotional needs of the disaffected young people who in the mid– to late 1960s migrated to their communities—as alternatives to health, mental health, and social services facilities which the young found threatening, demeaning, or unresponsive.

The founders of the first alternative services resembled the earlier settlement house workers in their idealism and humanitarianism. They differed in their commitment to the kind of participatory democracy which animated the civil rights, antiwar, youth, and women's movements of the 1960s.[2] These activist workers believed that, given time and space to do it, ordinary people could help themselves and one another to deal with the vast majority of problems in living that confronted them. They questioned the appropriateness of professional services which labeled or stigmatized those who came for help, and, in their own work, blurred or obliterated boundaries between staff and clients: A teenager who was panicky one night might counsel another the next. Determined to remain responsive to their clients' needs these early workers continually advocated for the social changes that would make individual change more possible.

In 1967 a handful of switchboards, drop–in centers, free clinics, and runaway houses served marginal young people in the "hip" neighborhoods of a few large cities. Today there are approximately 2,000 hotlines, over 200 runaway houses, and 400 free clinics. They have been organized by people of all ages, classes and ideologies in small towns, suburbs and rural areas, as well as in the large cities. In Prince George's, a suburban and rural Maryland county, for example, one of three hotlines receives 1,400 calls a month, one of two runaway houses gives shelter and intensive counseling to over 350 young people each year, and a single one of the county's nine drop–in centers provides 600 hours of individual therapy each month.[3]

In the early years, alternative services were preoccupied with responding to the immediate needs of their young clients—for emergency medical care, a safe place during a bad drug trip, or short–term housing. More recently, they have expanded and diversified. Drop–in centers work with the families and teachers of the teenagers who come to them as well as the young people themselves. Runaway houses have opened long–term residences and foster care programs for those who cannot return home or would otherwise be institutionalized; and free clinics and hotlines have helped begin specialized counseling services for other and older groups—women, gays, the elderly, etc.

In the 1970s, the alternative service model was adopted by people who identified new community needs. They created drug and alcohol counseling programs, rape crisis centers, shelters for battered women, peer counseling and street work projects, holistic health centers, home birthing services, and programs designed specifically for old people and particular ethnic minorities.

Many of these programs are now beginning to emphasize the role of diet, exercise and lifestyle in precipitating and preventing physical and emotional dysfunction and the relationship between stress and physical and emotional illness. Some are using the centuries old preventive medical techniques of Chinese medicine, yoga and herbalism, homeopathy, massage, and chiropractic, and such modern self–help techniques as biofeedback, guided imagery, and lifestyle counseling to help their clients to achieve physical and emotional balance. Increasingly, workers in alternative services are regarding these and other pyschophysical techniques as a natural complement to a system of care which emphasizes the whole person in a supportive environment, the ability of people to help themsleves and one another.

CHARACTERISTICS OF ALTERNATIVE SERVICES

Though alternative services are as diverse in their operation, staff and structure as their communities and clients, they share certain philosophical assumptions, attitudes, and practices which define their approach to mental health and illness as "alternative" and make them particularly useful and responsive to the people they serve. I have found the following to be among the most significant:

People's problems are responded to as those problems are experienced. A woman whose husband is beating her is regarded as a victim, not scrutinized as a masochist. A child who leaves his home is seen, housed, and fed as a runaway, not diagnosed as an acting–out disorder or judged to be a status offender. A man with chronic back pain and no demonstrable organic lesion is treated as a sufferer not dismissed as a malingerer.

Services are provided that are immediately accessible with a minimum of waiting and bureaucratic restriction. Hotlines, shelters for battered women, rape crisis centers, runaway houses, and many drop–in centers are open 24 hours a day, free to anyone who calls or comes in off the street.

Clients' problems are treated as signs of change and opportunities for growth rather than symptoms of an illness which must be suppressed. In drug–free alternatives to mental hospitalization such as San José California's Soteria, and Crossing Place in Washington, D.C., even psychotic episodes are regarded as potentially transformative and illuminating experiences.

Those who come to them for help are treated as members of families and social systems. This enables them to view their troubled clients' symptoms as reactions to and communications within their familial or social situation. It provides the underpinning for their treatment of pregnancy, childbirth, and dying primarily as shared family experiences and only secondarily, and occasionally, as medical conditions or emergencies. On a programmatic level this "systems" viewpoint encourages many alternative services to advocate for and work with their clients in the arena—job, home, school, or court—in which their problems arise.

Mental health professionals and the techniques they have developed are used but nonprofessionals are depended upon to deliver most of the primary care. In projects as diverse as runaway houses and home birth programs, free clinics and alternatives to mental hospitalization, professionals serve almost exclusively as consultants, trainers, and emergency back–up. They are there to share their knowledge with staff and clients and not necessarily to run the service.

Active client participation is regarded as the cornerstone of their mental health service program and indeed of mental health. On an individual therapeutic level this means emphasizing the strength of those who seek help and their capacity for self–help: Teenage runaways are encouraged to see themselves as potential agents for a family's change rather than helpless victims of its oppression, battered wives to become strong enough to leave rather than endure their husbands' brutality. In dozens of humanistic gerontology programs and in hundreds of free clinics and holistic healing centers, clients are encouraged to use techniques like biofeedback, progressive relaxation, acupressure, and guided imagery, and disciplines like Yoga and Tai Chi Chuan to experience, and then alter, physical and emotional states previously regarded as beyond their control.

On an organizational level this emphasis on self–help leads most alternative services to include present and former clients in their decision–making structure. It means devoting time and energy to creating formal and informal ways for those who have been helped to use their personal experience as a basis for helping others.

Both clients and staff are provided with a supportive and enduring community which transcends the delivery or receipt of a particular service. In a time when the extended family is losing its coherence and ties to hometowns and neighborhoods are fraying, alternative services are providing a continuing focus for collective allegience and an opportunity for long–term mutual support. For many who have long ago ceased to be official clients or workers they remain a retreat in times of trouble and a place to gather to celebrate joyous occasions.

The care provided is by any standards equal or superior to that offered by traditional mental health services. Many of the reports are anecdotal (i.e., the consistent finding that large numbers of young people with psychotic or borderline diagnoses are diverted from hospitalization by a variety of alternative services), but "harder" data is also beginning to accumulate: A two–year follow–up study of Soteria, a residential alternative to hospitalization funded by the National Institute of Mental Health, revealed that residents of the program "showed significantly better occupational levels and were more able to leave home to live independent of their families of origin" than a control group of people hospitalized on a crisis–oriented general hospital ward;[4] evaluation of S.A.G.E. (Senior Actualization and Growth Explorations) project in Berkeley has revealed striking psychological, cognitive, and physical improvements in the older people who participated in the program of gentle physical exercise, meditation, and group discussion;[5] and a matched population study of 1,046 home births and 1,046 hospital births has revealed significantly more infections and birth injuries in the group of babies that was delivered in the hospital.[6]

Generally, alternative services are more economical than the traditional services which their clients might otherwise use. Young people, many of whom come to runaway centers to avoid being hospitalized, provide an interesting example. In 1975 an NIMH study of 15 runaway centers around the country revealed that runaway centers spent from $32 to $50 a day for each young person housed; in contrast, the figures for acute care hospitalization ranged from $125 to $200 a day.[7] A more recent and sophisticated analysis of one runaway house, Someplace Else, in Tallahassee, Florida, revealed that this program was approximately three times as cost effective as the services routinely offered by the county. Long–term residential alternatives to hospitalization for adults like Soteria and the Training in Community Living program of the Mendota Mental Health Institute tend to be more expensive but here too cost–benefit analysis seems to reveal significant advantages for the alternative services.[8]

Alternative services have financial problems. The desire to work with whoever comes to them regardless of economic compensation, attempts to provide comprehensive and often unreimbursed services, unwillingness to take funds which restrict their work with clients, the complexity of Federal, State, and local funding procedures, and the general reluctance of many agencies to fund service programs that are neither certified by a professional establishment nor proven in scientific terms all conspire to keep most alternative services chronically underfunded.

Experience in trying to meet people's direct service needs can then become a basis for advocacy efforts on their clients' behalf. Hotlines which have noted an increase in a particular kind of problem—battered women, child abuse, etc.—have used their statistical information and their moral authority as service providers to prod local mental health and social service agencies to create programs to meet these needs. Groups which serve old people, pregnant women, and runaways have organized on a State and national level to advocate for legislation and funding to further and protect their clients' interests.

Changing and expanding the work they do to meet the changing needs of their clients is regarded as their responsibility. During the last several years centers for runaways have enlisted professionals to help them create family counseling programs. They have opened long–term residences and foster placement programs for young people who can't or won't go home; drop–in centers for teenagers who are having problems at home but don't want to leave their families; and educational, vocational, and health–care services to equip all of these young people to survive and deal with the adult world.

PROSPECTS FOR THE FUTURE

Many alternative services combine the skills and thoroughness of professionals with the commitment to service, responsiveness, and organizational flexibility of nonprofessionals. They are already providing effective, low–cost mental health services to large numbers—probably several millions—of Americans of all ages, races, and classes.[9] Any attempt to make mental health services more responsive to people's felt needs should take account of the kinds of programmatic innovations that alternative services have been making, of the new techniques being developed in holistic health practice, and of the spirit which pervades the entire alternative service movement.

Though some alternative services will function best when dealing with a particular problem or group, others may in the future evolve into new kinds of central places where troubled and troubling people could be offered comprehensive services. These new places could continue to be called community mental health centers, but they might better be called "human service centers," "community centers," or simply "centers." The names, designed to indicate a responsiveness to people's needs, would avoid creating the feelings of deprecation inevitably associated with describing oneself as "mentally ill."

Instead of spending the majority of their time seeing patients in their offices, professionals in these centers would largely devote themselves to a much expanded version of the "consultation and education" that is now so often neglected. Their primary job would be to consult with community people about the services they have already begun, and to catalyze, but not dominate, efforts to create new residential, counseling, and community development programs.

Rather than define problems in mental health terminology, center staff would help people to define their own problems in their own terms. If a woman with five children were suicidally depressed because of the inadequacy of her welfare payments, the dreariness of her home, and the rats that threaten her family, the center's crisis team would: work first of all on these realities: help her deal with the welfare department; assist her with child care; and bring in an exterminator. Instead of involving her in long–term psychotherapy or drug treatment, it might help her to become part of a support group of parents in similar situations. In the context of this group she might at some point feel free to talk about the personal problems which so many mental health professionals would insist on attacking first.

For people who needed them, various kinds of residences would be available. Thus someone experiencing the personality disintegration and overwhelming anxiety which often signal an acute psychotic episode would be able to go to a crisis house or to stay with a family where he or she could be guided and protected by a specially patient and skillful staff. These symptoms would not be suppressed by drugs. Instead the psychotic episode could become the kind of natural healing process that it is in some traditional societies and in such modern experimental communities as Soteria. Similarly, center workers might consult with or help start shelters for other groups—young people who could not live at home, "women in transition," or older individuals without social support—where these people could gain perspective on their lives and share their problems without defining themselves as mentally ill.

Though a dangerous and uncontrollable few would continue to require institutionalization, the vast majority of those who need longer term care could be kept in their own communities—in ordinary houses easily accessible to friends and relatives. Many of these people could— if staff workers provided organization and leadership—learn to take care of one another. Already some shelters for battered women and residences for older teenagers are run by clients; certainly old people who are healthy but homeless could supervise the care of young people who are chronically ill; and students at colleges or young workers could be subsidized—well below the cost of conventional foster care—to live with runaways who lack homes to which they could return.

The majority of people with problems do not, of course, need crisis intervention or residential services. Instead of assuming they needed therapy, centers would offer them the resources—professional expertise, advocacy, and education—to help them deal with their own problems. People would be helped to understand themselves as actually suffering from life crises, and as members of a family, office, work group, or class. Techniques of family counseling, group therapy, and community organizing could be used to help make the family, class-room, or work place more responsive to all its participants, giving them the tools to continue to work things out long after the center workers withdraw.

At the same time, some centers might begin to provide the kind of ongoing individualized health care which has been lacking in our society. Under the supervision of physicians who are developing a holistic perspective on health and mental health, physician's assistants, nurse practitioners, and neighborhood people trained by them could discuss and review each person's physical and emotional well–being, and could investigate the economic, occupational, familial, and in-trapsychic causes of stress in their lives. Together they could formulate a regime of diet, exercise, and relaxation, or help them to look for other employment, more education, or different housing.

Groups of people with special concerns or problems—women wanting to share with each other questions about their roles as women; parents of retarded or autistic children; old people wishing to improve their psychological and physical functioning—would be helped, as needed, to form groups with or without a leader in which they could discuss and deal with their common concerns.

Individual therapy would still be available, but there would be a shift in emphasis toward helping people to develop the capacity to analyze their social situations and physical and emotional needs and thus be able to use a network of helpers both within the center and outside. The biological aspect of their treatment would also change: instead of relying on drugs to elevate mood or calm anxiety, to deaden headaches or stop gastric secretion, people would be taught to deal with these conditions through biofeedback, meditation, yoga, acu-pressure, Tai Chi, and massage. Learning to use these self–help tech-niques would enable people to avoid prolonged dependency on professional helpers, contribute to their sense of control over their own lives, and remove the possibility of dangerous side effects and diminished performance which always attend the use of psychotropic drugs.

This kind of center could be a continuing source of the kinds of primary prevention programs that the mental health establishment often talks of but rarely spends time and money to bring about. To-gether, staff and clients of the center could help other agencies develop education, recreation, and community action programs, and campaign for more responsive policies in the institutions which affect people's lives—from welfare offices to hospitals to factories. For the community as a whole, the center—which would have clients on its governing board—would be the kind of gathering place that alternative services already are, a place where people could come when they wanted to help as well as be helped, when they just felt like being with others, as well as when they were in trouble.

Any attempt to make the kinds of changes herein described will require a different attitude, a new kind of training—not only of the physicians, psychologists, and social workers who will help facilitate this change but of the paraprofessionals and the clients with whom they will work. Professionals need training which helps them to understand how their attitudes and convictions are formed by their own values and culture, and how these may at times prevent them from working effectively with other people. They also need to learn that in addition to being bearers of knowledge and purveyors of new techniques, they are the servants of those for whom they work. At the same time, community people who crave a common purpose and some larger goal will have the opportunity to learn and use new skills.

In the context of a participatory healing community, the boundaries between helpers and helped will blur and the very nature of mental health work will be transformed. Even the most arduous tasks may well change their character: for most attendants, the experience of working with mad people in a hospital setting is grim, demeaning, and uncomfortable; working with the same people in a place like Soteria or in one of the group foster homes that I have helped develop is, though exhausting, enormously exciting and challenging.

CONCLUSION

The point of all this is not simply to produce another kind of treatment, or another kind of professional, and certainly not to insist that all centers do all things in a particular way, but to change the structure of treatment and the delivery of services; to relate to troubled people on their terms; to insist that their needs—not the preconceptions or self–interest of any professional group—shape the kind of help they receive; to give them the opportunity to use their full potential to heal themselves; and to support and enlarge—not usurp—the kinds of initiatives that alternative services have already taken. None of the reforms I have proposed is Utopian, and all of them together will not, of course, create a Utopia, but they are a start, a step toward relieving at least some to the human misery that we have too complacently and too long regarded as the symptoms of mental illness.

REFERENCES

1. Bryant, T. *Preliminary report of the President's commission on mental health.* September 1, 1977.
2. Gordon, J.S. Coming together: Consultation with young people. *Social Policy,* July–August 1974.
3. Statistics gathered by the Special Study on Alternative Services. James S. Gordon, M.D., Director for the President's Commission on Mental Health, 1978.
4. Mosher, L.R., & Menn, A.Z. *Community residential treatment for schizophrenia: Two year follow–up data.* Unpublished, 1977.
5. Lieberman, M. Personal communication. University of Chicago, 1978.
6. Mehl, L.E. Research on alternatives in child birth: What can it tell us about hospital practice. *Twenty–first Century Obstetrics,* NAPSAC, 1977.
7. Gordon, J.S. *Alternative services: A recommendation for public funding.* Unpublished, 1975.
8. Weisbrod, B.A., Test, M.A., & Stein, L.I. *An alternative to the mental hospital—benefits and costs.* Unpublished, 1977.
9. Gordon, J.A. *Final Report of the Special Study on Alternative Services to the President's Commission on Mental Health, February 1978.*

Chapter 19

THE WHOLE SOCIETY: MEDICINE IN AN UNHEALTHY WORLD

Rick J. Carlson, J.D.

Much of what is in this volume is new; some is rediscovered. It represents the "health renaissance" we have been experiencing in the United States in recent years and is, in part, the result of a growing disenchantment with aspects of traditional medicine. Some of the contributors to this volume argue for wider access to many of the techniques and modalities which represent this "renaissance." I wonder if this is desirable; if all or most, or even some of these new approaches to health should be "integrated" into the medicine generally available to everyone?

This large question harbors many others: Do we know enough to argue for or against integration? What about the safety, efficacy, and effectiveness of these new approaches?; What about minimal training and educational requirements for practitioners?; What about third–party reimbursement? These are controversial, often heated issues. To some, the whole integral medicine or holistic health is suspect. To others it represents the only hope for further gains in health. The truth probably lies somewhere between the extremes. I would like to explore some of the major public policy issues that are raised by the question of integration and some of the key ideas about health and illness that will in turn shape policy decisions.

A Short History of Ideas

In the early 1800s, memories of the plagues were not far distant. Population size and food supply were steadily increasing. The infectious diseases were the major killers, but the rates of such diseases had already begun a slow decline which was to continue into this century. There was a medicine already more systematic than much of its shamanistic roots, but still lacking a method of inquiry. Traditional Judeo–Christian beliefs held that the responsibility for health was largely outside the individual; it rested on the nature of the relationship between the person and God, and depended more on God's beneficence than human agency. In the last decades of the nineteenth century there were two critical developments: First, the scientific method became generally known and its application to the practice of medicine served as a means of transforming the idiosyncracies of practice and the ungrounded assumptions upon which they rested into a more systematic science. Second, perceived relationships between certain environmental factors such as water quality and the health levels of persons exposed to particular environmental factors prompted the initiation of massive public health programs. These two developments, based on a common epistemology—of cause–effect relationships— were major steps toward the medicine of today.

In the early 1900s our society had some fundamental health–care options. What evidence there is suggests that the principal gains in human health prior to the beginnings of the century were achieved through nontherapeutic methods, principally public–health measures, and through improvements in the quality and amount of food. Yet at the same time therapeutic medicine was gaining ascendance. This seeming anomaly may be in part attributed to the availability of a scientific method which made it possible to draw causal relationships between therapeutic interventions and outcomes to patients. More importantly, therapeutic medicine was gaining in political and economic strength as the number of its practitioners increased. The Flexner report, issued in 1910, insured the preeminence of therapeutic medicine as it led to near monopolistic control by allopathic medicine over the institutions of health.

Thus by the beginning of the century we as a society had chosen to emphasize the identification, management, and extirpation of the agents of disease instead of focusing on and amplifying programs designed to improve the quality of the environment and to further strengthen the human host.

The results of that choice have been significant. We have gained considerable information about human biology, and we have learned much about the means of curing and treating illness. It wasn't necessarily the wrong choice, and of course much biomedical research still needs to be undertaken. We are now, however, poised for a fundamental change in perspective—a change which may restore social, environmental, and behavioral factors to the influential position in shaping health policy which the evidence about their relationship to health has always demanded. What follows are some of the health policy implications of this almost inevitable change in perspective.

THE SCOPE OF MEDICAL PRACTICE: CAN THE DOCTOR BE NUTRITIONIST, TOO?

In recent years the push towards a holistic perspective on health has faced even sympathetic physicians with a dilemma. Many thoughtful physicians recognize that there are many aspects of health for which their training never prepared them. Moreover, most acknowledge the critical importance of environmental and behavioral factors, nearly all of which lie beyond the scope of modern medical training. Under these circumstances, there are some who argue that as a matter of public policy, physicians, and other health professionals should be trained to understand better the roles played by the environmental and behavioral determinants of health. Many argue, more strongly, that the physician is so limited in his or her understanding of health that the education of the health professional must necessarily be broadened.

On the other hand, there are those who argue that the burden of medical education is already so great that to broaden it would place intolerable pressures on the student. Instead of training physicians in environmental and behavioral sciences they would rather intensify physician's training as technicians to meet the needs of already ill. Arguing that great technical skill and expertise are required for those health problems which cannot or have not been prevented, they suggest other health professionals be trained to deal with the other determinants of health requiring attention. Such a step was taken recently in California when medical schools were asked to propose budgets which reduced the cost of medical education. Their response was to

propose a medical curriculum with diminished information about nutrition, a subject that has traditionally been excluded from biomedical
education.

A movement to restrict the scope of medical education may, of
course, fail to resolve a number of other critical policy issues. While
many physicians, and indeed, organized medicine itself, are sympathetic to the need to train other health professionals and to create
public programs to influence the health levels of populations along
environmental and behavioral lines, they remain loathe to part with
any of the money they get for medical practice. This resource allocation
issue dwarfs strong evidence that environmental and behavioral interventions are more likely to improve our health than continued ex-
penditures for medical care, further complicating any discussion of
the scope of medical education.

Finally, as long as physicians continue to monopolize health care,
health–professional education emphasizing behavioral and environmental considerations is not likely to attract the same caliber of students
as medical education. Moreover, unless health professionals who are
trained in the environmental and behavioral area have equal statute
in the health–care system, these areas are likely to continue to be
shortchanged in future resource allocation decisions.

THE DIFFERENCE BETWEEN TECHNIQUE AND CONCEPT

The discussing the "integration" of holistic practice into conventional medicine one must take into account the critical stance that many
physicians have adopted towards the techniques they associate with
"holism." Many of them seem to think that holistic medicine is nothing
more than a little acupuncture or Chinese medicine, a little biofeedback, some esoteric bodywork techniques—mostly developed in California, and applied there as well—and equally exotic nutritional
practices,—all overlaid by dubious psychological counseling. Such an
interpretation trivializes the concept.

The term "holistic," first coined by Jan Smuts in 1926, has come
to be applied to almost every aspect of human behavior. Smuts' original
use of the word was epistemological. To Smuts the prevailing "reductionist" perspective resulted in an unrelenting of the parts of systems without consideration of how those parts interacted in larger
systems and without consideration, or even acknowledgment, of phenomena which represented more than the sum of any set of parts.
Hence, holistic thinking in its original and fullest sense was an antidote
to the reductionist epistemology underlying modern scientific thought.

In recent years the word "holistic" has been widely applied in both medicine and health. Used in several different ways, the first and least important is the application of the term to a variety of "new" or rediscovered therapeutic modalities. Hence, the term is often applied to biofeedback practice, acupuncture, such bodywork therapies as the Feldenkrais technique and Rolfing, and other new approaches. Though practitioners of the healing arts may well be holistic in their orientation—that is to say, they may perceive and interact with their clients in a holistic way—the modalities themselves are no more inherently holistic than coronary artery bypass surgery. In this context holistic health is sometimes in danger of becoming a banner underneath which parade a variety of practitioners of various healing arts, some efficacious and some not, seeking the legitimation that the concept of holism ostensibly confers.

The term "holistic health" may also be applied to a political movement. In California and in some other parts of this country, the holistic health movement is a constituency with political as well as therapeutic objectives. According to my reading of history, traditional medicine gained its current ascendancy through political stratagems, not through the inarguable superiority of its therapeutic impact. It is not surprising then that practitioners made pariahs by medicine, and consumers whose dissatisfaction with traditional medicine is acute may find political agitation expedient. Certainly in California, where holistic practitioners are legion and where the number of consumers interested in holistic practices is large and growing, those associating themselves with holistic health form a constituency with real political leverage. There is nothing inherently wrong with with using the holistic perspective as a means to force fresh air into the practice of medicine. This is not, however, its more profound application.

The real power of holistic thinking lies in the perspective it brings to our perception of who we are as human beings. Reductionist thinking in all fields, including medicine, results in the compartmentalization of the human being and human experience into those aspects or parts which are amenable to detailed analysis and/or intervention. This is the basic premise of the prevailing medical model. Though it has its utility, it is a profoundly limited view of human beings. Holistic thinking as an epistemological notion requires that the human being be perceived as a whole person made up of physiological, emotional, intellectual, and spiritual dimensions that dynamically interact. Any approach to improving the health of human beings, either as individuals or in groups, will require placing them in a larger and richer context than medicine typically offers.

This shift towards the holistic perspective is really irreversible, not because it is being forced upon medicine so urgently, but rather because it is part of a much larger change in perspective about who and what we are as humans. Its application to medicine is just one aspect of a more embracing paradigm shift which affects and is apparent in the theory and practice of post–Einsteinian physics and in the complex and shifting interrelationships of such diverse fields as ecology and international and transnational problem solving.

THE EPISTEMOLOGY OF PRACTICE: BELIEF AND RESULT

The concept of responsibility involves the belief that people "choose" their sickness and its form, and the conviction—as articulated most powerfully by Carl and Stephanie Simonton[1] in discussions of their work with cancer patients—that the patients' beliefs and motivation will significantly affect the outcome of their illness. This point of view differs radically from the premises of conventional medical practice which hold that disease is something that is either indiscriminate, governed by a person's constitution, or secondary to inherent weaknesses or recent debility, and that its successful treatment is largely in the physician's hands.

This fundamental difference in perspective will have to be dealt with in any attempt to integrate traditional and holistic medicine. It is clear that if you approach a sick individual with the assumption that he or she has somehow "chosen" to be ill, the therapeutic approach you recommend will necessarily be very different than if you believe that the illness was beyond his or her responsibility.

MONEY AND TRUTH: THE ORIGINS OF MODERN MEDICINE

At a recent talk I gave to a group of physicians at a California Medical Association meeting, I asked them to imagine themselves in the same room at the turn of the century. I told them that if we had all been there 79 years ago about every third person in the room would have been a homeopath. I reminded them that the practice of medicine prior to 1910 was mixed; a variety of medical theories including homeopathy and allopathy competed. Yet, in the years from 1900 to 1920 homeopathy was driven underground. One interpretation of this is the superior therapeutic efficacy of allopathic practice, the theory upon which modern medicine is based, simply won the day. Other sources including Harris Coulter's *The Divided Legacy*[2] suggest otherwise. The evidence they present demonstrates that the virtual disappearance of homeopathy had more to do with the economic and political power of allopathic practitioners than with its therapeutic failures.

Indeed, the question of integration is less likely to be resolved on the basis of therapeutic efficacy than on the basis of economic and political power. Under these circumstances, holistic practitioners—the power of the concept of holism notwithstanding—are at a decided disadvantage. If the medical establishment chooses to suppress holistic practice, it may well succeed, if history is any guide, widespread belief in holistic practices notwithstanding. Though this does not preclude some limited amount of integration nor a drift of philosophical orientation in the direction of holism, it does suggest that the expectation that holistic practice will overcome allopathic practice is unrealistic.

Conclusion

Even if its technical and institutional manifestations are not yet clearly evident, the holistic idea—and perspective—is one whose time has come. Because the premises of existing practice are strong and pervasive and will compete with holistic or integral medicine, however, a radical transformation of medical practice is unlikely. Moreover, the political and economic, and even the social and cultural strength of the current system will continue to outstrip a competing holistic system. This does not weaken the idea of holism, but simply means that the idea must find its way into institutional practice over time. In fact, if holistic practices were immediately integrated into existing practice, the result would most likely be the impoverishment of holistic practices rather than the enrichment of conventional practice.

The power of the holistic approach to health and healing is that service providers view their patients or clients as whole persons, and themselves as guides helping individuals find the routes (and metaphors) that make sense for them. The patient or client, unwilling to accept a narrow technological approach to a complex human problem, fully participates in this process. It is very difficult to translate this rich interpersonal experience into reimbursable units of services in the same manner as injections, surgical procedures, or drugs. Though some diagnostic and therapeutic holistic practices, such as biofeedback and biological analyses, can be successfully and realistically integrated into conventional practice, most of what is rich about the holistic orientation must necessarily remain outside the fee–for–service reimbursement medical care system. Attempts to integrate the perspective, as it translates into practice, may erode the practice, and in turn, vitiate the perspective.

The holistic perspective is here to stay, and though some of its practices can be made more widely available through the existing health care delivery system, much of what is important and, in the long run, powerful about holism, will and must remain outside of any medical–care system—a part of the way we live rather than an item in any scheme of health care.

REFERENCES

1. Simonton, C., Matthews-Simonton, S. & Creighton, J. *Getting well again*, Los Angeles: Tarcher, 1978.
2. Coulter, Harris, *The divided legacy*. Washington, D.C.: Wehawken Book Co. Vol. I, 1975; Vol. II, 1976; Vol. III, 1977.

Appendix:

A RESOURCE GUIDE TO INTEGRAL MEDICINE

compiled by
David E. Bresler, Ph.D.
Dennis T. Jaffe, Ph.D.
James S. Gordon, M.D.

1. Center for Integral Medicine
    P.O. Box 967
    Pacific Palisades, California 90272

   A nonprofit educational organization founded in 1974 by a group of health professionals who wished to shift the perspective of health care from the diagnosis and treatment of illness to the development and maintenance of health and life. The Center offers an extensive series of professional and public training programs, published reports, pamphlets, tapes, and other educational materials, and sponsors periodic conferences and symposia.

2. Institute for Noetic Sciences
    600 Stockton Street
    San Francisco, California 94108

   A research and educational institute which funds various projects concerning integral medicine and the nature of consciousness. The

Institute's publications include a bibliography of integral medicine and reports of projects on cancer, aging, homeopathy, super healthy people, and other related areas. IONS also publishes a newsletter and sponsors periodic conferences.

3. Holistic Health Organizing Committee
    P.O. Box 166
    Berkeley, California 94703

Stresses preventive medicine and health education as well as full recognition and legal protection for all forms of alternative healing and their qualified practitioners. Sponsors a newsletter and programs on the legal aspects of holistic health approaches.

4. The East West Academy of Healing Arts
    Council of Nurse Healers
    60 Ora Way
    San Francisco, California 94131

Dedicated to expanding the existing body of knowledge relevent to healing modalities in nursing through theory development, research, and practice. EWAHA provides a communication and education network for nurses and the community at large.

5. Association for Holistic Health
    P.O. Box 33202
    San Diego, California 92103

A nonprofit educational corporation dedicated to promoting and supporting holistic health and to ensuring its continued development in professional methods, standards, and ethics. AHH is involved in the development of a model holistic health center, publishes its annual *Journal of Holistic Health*, and sponsors an annual conference.

6. Hawaii Health Net
    2535 South King Street
    Honolulu, Hawaii 96814

A communications network to assist individuals in finding viable alternatives to personal health care.

7. American Holistic Medical Association
    6932 Little River Turnpike
    Annandale, Virginia 22003

A professional membership organization for physicians interested in an alternative to the AMA. AHMA publishes a professional journal and sponsors periodic training programs and conferences.

8. The East/West Center for Holistic Health
    275 Madison Avenue, Suite 500
    New York, New York 10016

Dedicated to promoting effective approaches to total health and wholeness with the recognition of mind–body–spirit unity. EWCHH sponsors conferences and is developing a holistic health facility.

9. Society for Wholistic Medicine
    137 South Garfield Avenue
    Hinsdale, Illinois 60521

Publishes a series of monographs concerning the development, implementation, and evaluation of church–based, university–medical–center–sponsored health centers. They also have published a report on the national health conference they sponsor along with the Kellogg Foundation.

10. Family Health Foundation
     3733 Oliver, N.W.
     Washington, D.C. 20015

A nonprofit educational and research group directed by James S. Gordon, M.D. particularly concerned with training families and non-physician health care providers in health promotion and natural first aid, and with helping physicians to integrate alternative healing techniques—acupuncture, meditation, nutrition, osteopathic manipulation, homeopathy—into their practices.

11. New Directions in Medicine
     Suite 1200
     1140 Connecticut Ave N.W.
     Washington, D.C. 20036

A directory and clearinghouse of educational opportunities for medical students and residents. A book of the same name listing the 180 participating preceptors and resource persons is available from Aurora Associates.

Part II: Newsletters and Magazines Related to Integral Medicine

1. *Brain Mind Bulletin*
   Interface Press
   P.O. Box 42211
   Los Angeles, California 90042

The Bulletin, edited by Marilyn Ferguson, covers research, conferences, events, books, and all manner of useful information for researchers, clinicians, and interested laymen.

2. *Holistic Health Review*
   Holistic Health Organizing Committee
   1030 Merced Street
   Berkeley, California 94707

Formed by a coalition of Bay Area health services, this review offers articles, interviews, reviews, and policy information.

3. *Medical Self–Care*
   Box 717
   Inverness, California 94937

MSC focuses on methods of self–help used to maintain health, with practical columns, reviews of relevant material, resources and classes, and how-to information. It is edited by Tom Ferguson whose principle is that the best care is self–care. Past issues have focused on women's health, children, jogging, stress, and the use of personal journals.

4. *Journal of Holistic Health*
   Association for Holistic Health
   P.O. 33202
   San Diego, California 92103

The Association's Journal contains transcripts edited from the proceedings of their yearly conferences, held in San Diego in the first week in September.

5. *Somatics*
   1516 Grant Avenue, Suite 220
   Novato, California 94947

A new magazine edited by Tom Hanna that focuses on the bodily arts and sciences, including health, psychophysiology, ecology, and philosophical issues.

6. *Common Sense*
   Commonweal
   Box 316
   Bolinas, California 94924

Quarterly newsletter focused on environmental health issues and health policy.

7. *Harvard Medical School Health Letter*
   79 Garden Street
   Cambridge, Massachusetts 02138

Provides nontechnical information concerning various illnesses, diseases, and medical problems for consumers.

8. *New Age*
   P.O. Box 4921
   Manchester, New Hampshire 03108

This magazine covers all aspects of the new consciousness movement, including its political and social implications. It contains many columns, ads, and current events. The May 1978 issue was on holistic health.

9. *New Realities*
   P.O. Box 26289
   San Francisco, California 94126

Formerly *Psychic Magazine*, the focus is on paranormal phenomena and consciousness, east and west.

10. *Prevention*
    33 East Minor Street
    Emmaus, Pennsylvania 18049

This is one of the most widely read health and nutrition magazines, offering articles on health, the value of foods, vitamins, and the role of nutrition in healing.

11. *Life and Health*
         6856 Eastern Avenue, N.W.
         Washington, D.C. 20012

After 93 years, this publication still offers short informative articles on general aspects of health and health care.

12. *Human Behavior*
         12031 Wilshire Boulevard
         Los Angeles, California 90025

This magazine includes reviews of journal articles, general articles covering all aspects of behavior, and interviews with noted social scientists.

13. *Human Nature*
         P.O. Box 9110
         Greenwich, Connecticut 06830

This new magazine on human sciences could be described as a cross between *Scientific American* and *Psychology Today*.

14. *East West Journal*
         P.O. Box 305
         Dover, New Jersey 07801

This magazine/journal contains feature articles, columns, ads, and a classified section, with a strong emphasis on health care.

15. *Medical Research Bulletin*
         A.R.E. Clinic
         4018 North 40th Street
         Phoenix, Arizona 85018

Based on the writings of psychic Edgar Cayce, the Bulletin is edited by William McGarey, M.D., and contains case histories, news notes and abstracts from the medical literature.

16. *Natural Bulletin*
         Notre 59A at Brookhill Drive
         West New York, New York 10994

Edited by Carlson Wade, this newsletter contains feature columns, self–help quizzes, health times, and consumer information.

17. *National Health Federation Bulletin*
     212 West Foothill Boulevard
     Monrovia, California 91016

This bulletin "serves its readers as a forum for the presentation of minority or conflicting points of view, rather than by publishing only material on which a consensus has been reached."

18. *Nutrition and the M.D.*
     7060 Hollywood Boulevard, Suite 726
     Hollywood, California 90028

This highly technical newsletter contains brief summaries of nutrition research studies, questions and answers, new products, and reference sources for professionals.

PART III. PRIVATELY CIRCULATED EDUCATIONAL MATERIALS

Many of the preceding organizations publish monographs and reports concerning various areas of integral medicine. In addition, here are selected educational materials which are highly recommended.

1. Center for Integral Medicine
    P.O. Box 967
    Pacific Palisades, California 90272

In cooperation with UCLA School of Medicine and UCLA Extension, the Center has produced a large series of self–study educational programs, consisting of comprehensive workbooks, cassette tapes of lectures and experiential exercises, and self–study materials and examinations. These can be taken on an independent study basis for continuing education credit for physicians, nurses, and other health professionals. Courses include "An Introduction to Integral Medicine," "Fundamentals of Biofeedback," "New Frontiers in Pain Control," "Clinical Hypnotherapy," "Stress Management in Clinical Practice," and others. Write for catalogue.

2. Wellness Workbook
    Wellness Associates
    42 Miller Avenue
    Mill Valley, California 94941

John Travis studied community medicine and public health at the Johns Hopkins University, then decided to create a wellness center that would not treat sickness but would help people to increase their level of wellness. Travis and his colleagues have designed a self–help workbook containing a self–assessment of health as well as information on how to increase wellness. Also available is a professional health–care kit.

3. Himalayan International Institute
    RD1
    Honesdale, Pennyslvania 18421

The Institute publishes a series of books integrating Yoga with Western medicine and psychotherapy. *Yoga and Psychotherapy*, a hardcover book by Institute staff Swami Rama, Swami Ajaya, and Dr. R. Ballentine is a synthesis of Western and Eastern knowledge organized around the chakras. The Institute also conducts training programs and holds a conference on yoga and meditation in June of each year.

4. Learning for Health
    1314 Westwood Boulevard
    Los Angeles, California 90024

This group publishes a self–help workbook to teach the skills of maintaining health, as well as tapes, articles, and other materials for health professionals. These materials can be used in clinics and medical settings to promote more effective psychosocial interventions and patient self–care. It is directed by Dennis T. Jaffe, Ph.D.

5. Stress, Psychological Factors, and Cancer
    Cancer Counseling and Research Center
    1413 8th Avenue
    Fort Worth, Texas 76104

The Center has published an annotated bibliography of research into stress factors and the psychology of cancer, documenting the scientific basis of the Simontons' therapeutic program. It includes summaries of each article and an extensive bibliography, as well as their emerging model concerning the psychophysiology of cancer. Also available from CCRC is a research paper, "Psychology of the Exceptional Cancer Patient: A Description of Patients who Outlive Predicted Life Expectancies" and other articles and tapes about the Simontons' work, including their book, *Getting Well Again*.

6. Selective Awareness
     1230 University Drive
     Menlo Park, California 94025

Emmett Miller, M.D. has prepared a workbook, articles, and a large number of cassette tapes combining meditation, hypnotic induction, and music. These can be used in a self–healing and personal–change program.

INDEX